Will the Real Healer Please Stand Up

Impossible Healing in the Blink of an Eye

The Neuroscience
of
Spontaneous Healing

Knowing Thyself.

Including

Medical, Neuroscience, NLP & Coaching Plus Support Healing as a More Powerful Combined Therapy.

Following
Activating Spontaneous Healing published 2007

by
Robert P. Denton

Edition: Oxford English 23/08/2017

Discover case histories of "Therapeutic Healing," which demonstrate powerful links between Medical, Neuroscience, NLP, coaching, intuition, telepathy, emotional intelligence and a raft of brain intelligence centres.

Faith and spiritual healing are steeped in centuries of mystique and come in a multitude of forms and shapes with no real understanding of why they came into being or how they might give the appearance of working.

In the entire science of healing be it orthodox doctors and surgeons, registered therapies or alternative forms of healing, none of these have ever healed anyone in the entire history of mankind. If there is a paradox it is that the supposed healer is not the healer. This explanation is set on the basis of neuro and medical science, therefore this book aims to explain why this is the case. This account shows why some experienced doctors or surgeons understand the real healer is the innate healing intelligence of the person being healed.

What you need to know and do to activate your inner healer or innate healing intelligence.

When you learn how – When you are ready
Healing can be fascinating and fast.

1st Edition 17 August 2017

Cover design by Robert P. Denton   -

The Peony takes its name from the mythological Greek character Paeon, who studied with Asclepius the God of medicine but actually a demigod, born of a divine father, Apollo, and a mortal mother, Coronis.

Published by FirstHousePress

THE TRUTH IS NOT FOR EVERYONE
ONLY FOR THOSE WHO SEEK IT

Whatever we do in life there is one fundamental favour we all can do that is vital to our inner wellbeing and success.

"To Thine Own Self be True"

Disclaimer and Copyright Notice

Contents

You Are The Healer

Healer Heal Thyself
and then you will know the
Impossible Happens in the Blink of an Eye.

Healing begins in knowing thyself.

Why life coaching and NLP are powerful healing therapies

by
Robert P. Denton

The Neuroscience of Spontaneous Healing.

Insights into how to help re-activate
the innate healing system.

For further information about the power of the mind go to:
www.neurofaultprotection.com

Introduction

YOU ARE THE HEALER

An inscription on the Greek temple at Delphi said, *"Know thyself and thou shall know all the mysteries of the gods and of the universe?"*

Plato said, *"To know the universe first know thyself. To know thyself first know your mind."*

To *"know thyself"* may first of all have been simply a warning not to pay attention to gossip or the opinions of the multitudes. Later on "Knowing thyself" became an important part of discovering how to achieve one's best. Throughout our lives the more we know ourselves the better chance we have to succeed in all we aspire to. Knowing thyself and activating your own innate healing system when it is thrown off balance or gets stuck, has a great deal to do with self confidence and good personal leadership. Whether you are flying with success or the chips are down, knowing thyself, self confidence and good personal leadership are vital to both, doing even better or sorting a mess out with minimal if no further mistakes or stress. When we are grounded to face an unexpected challenge, the more we know ourselves the more we have trust in our self-leadership. The less we know of ourselves the more likely to consciously limit our own potential to succeed by knee jerk reactions and poor, if not bad decisions.

What we believe to be true and valid influences all we allow ourselves to think and therefore how we support or limit our own imagination, and creativity, thus we grow or block our own potential. Depending on the beliefs and values we chose to aspire to, they determine whether our thinking and therefore our performance is continually spiralling upwards or whether conforming to the average status quo of a ho-hum lifestyle of mediocrity or worst into the depths of impoverished thinking.

Limited self knowledge restricts development and the capability to push perceived boundaries of performance especially when under pressure. Horses for courses, is; about knowing the truth of ourselves, which helps to focus on what we are naturally good at and therefore what skills to develop, thus also which lifestyle or professional direction to take. Working with ourselves in this way helps to maintain inner harmony and therefore life is less of a struggle. Knowing ourselves goes far beyond school or professional performance, it helps us to better manage all the smaller aches and pains of life also how to overcome them quickly and easily. Knowing thyself helps us to know if we are just having an off day or whether there is something internally or emotionally that needs a little more or frankly a lot more attention.

As far as this book is concerned, "One man's meat is another man's poison." What is good for others may not be good for ourselves, relates to guiding us to know ourselves, our weaknesses and susceptibilities sufficiently to stay away from what can damage us, our performance or our hopes, dreams, our aspirations and indeed our life.

As you will further discover as these chapters unravel, the human brain, mind body are a conglomerate of incredible centres of intelligence. Like everything in nature, nothing is 100% perfect. So, "A stitch in time saves nine" is knowing thyself as a quick reference to nipping health and emotional problems in the bud before a minor molehill becomes a challenging mountain of nagging health stresses silently undermining your best efforts.

Clearly good psychological and physical health is of prime importance to a happy, successful and active life. These things are necessary for balanced and performance in whatever we do. Yet our habitual box of perceptions or psychological parameters, belief limitations, and our values, all of, which we use daily to manage our lives; may hide both good, not so good and positively unhelpful subconscious limiting behaviours.

We are not alone, there is help at hand. Psychometric tests are designed to see through the smoke and mirrors we use to accidentally or deliberately hide our perceived or real imperfections also to embellish the capabilities we claim to excel in. These are mainly employed by companies as an independent and speedy way to understand who each of their prospective employees really are. But psychometric tests are also extremely useful for our own development also balance of health. This is provided we can accept a level of pragmatic honesty, not quite so flattering as our alter ego would have us believe. Used wisely psychometric tests may guide us towards our ideal life style, what we are best suited to, which changes would improve our successes and thus unhelpful habits, which need to be checked. Look deeper and we see indications of how we think about ourselves. Closer inspection may reveal how we care for ourselves, also what this means in real terms of recognising how a given level of health and stress relates to personal performance.

Most people accept that prevention is always better than cure. How many actually follow this advice? This is so important when it comes to the important issue of emotional balance and therefore performance with less stress. If not constantly working at examining and improving our limiting thoughts, behaviours and health weaknesses that deplete our strengths- relative to our objectives, then life is going to be a greater struggle than it needs be. Good management of all these issues helps us to push the envelope in whatever subject or direction we want, particularly when we want it. One of the most important issues is doing this while keeping unnecessary stress under a firm control.

The mention of stress, intuition, telepathy and non-interference are going to appear frequently in this book because they are connected to so many health conditions and performance. Therefore, they are also important to healing support and innate spontaneous healing.

Stress is something I made a particular point of studying after my own stress burnout crisis in and around 1995. Apart from the effects of stress, burnout was a wakeup call for me signalling how out of balance my life was. It was more than 90% focused on business and less than10% given over to caring for myself and the remainder of my life and objectives. The fact is that my personal objectives became completely sidelined and essentially forgotten. When Burnout happened it was all too late. The greater personal tragedy and paradox of this was that within this side of my life I was assisting other people to find a better balance in their own lives. Ooops!

A fairly average easy going person may miss simple things like taking notice of how they feel in themselves and are they anywhere near achieving all or any of their goals. For example: if we feel well, we are well and we do well but do we actively take advantage of that feel-good state to do even better? If we do not feel well and that feel-good sensation we hear others talking about seems to have escaped us, why is that, what have we missed? Good business management constantly keeps an eye on how well their company performance is. Since we are our personal CEO, we should be faced with the same questions of how well are we actually doing? Are we doing and achieving what we set our hearts on or have we been side-tracked into a substandard or impoverished version. Indeed, are we doing better than we had ever dreamed of? - How can we develop that and use it elsewhere in our lives? - What are we? - Who are we? - What have we become by purposeful design of adequate caring or by default of not knowing ourselves and thus not caring enough for what we are really capable of doing?

When we are doing well we tend to ignore warning signs of things to come. When we are in prime condition to throw ourselves into doing greater things, we may forget about the most important thing – balance. Those who take notice of these things will have noticed that life tends to move in cycles of harmony and easy performance followed by periods of disruptive disharmony. These chaotic periods eventually revert to harmony and easy performance before moving into the next cycle of disharmony. During the disharmony is when we are most susceptible to making unnecessary mistakes and causing ourselves avoidable stress. The worse the disharmony and chaos, the more we have likely given little or no attention to forward planning during the periods of harmony and balance.

Being consciously aware we are firing on all cylinders with a clear mind, should be a good day to have the initiative and confidence to successfully push performance boundaries in ways we had not considered possible before. This may be something new or the time to do something we have been continually putting off because it is a bit of a stretch. For the majority of us these good-high-potential-performance days have a limited shelf life and when they are over we may have to dig deep in our performance resources just to keep on track. Therefore the better we know ourselves, the better we can care for ourselves in the best way possible for our greater performance at all times and in all situations. If we feel under par, then our thinking suffers. As a result our general health, immune system, performance and enjoyment of life suffer too. This may seem something of a lottery but only if we ignore latent skills of intuition and telepathy. When we are in touch with ourselves we will notice feelings or intuitive awareness that something unbalanced is heading our way. People who take notice of themselves in this way are alerted to not be caught off guard. They are extra careful during off-colour days or periods and take more notice of their inner feeling or intuitive guidance. Therefore they have a greater chance of avoiding mistakes while re-energising themselves for better times.

Better personal, health and career performance may be supported by NLP and life coaching. These disciplines are all part of the wider subject of neuroscience for the reason they help us to better know how our minds function. The greatest gifts self awareness and knowing ourselves bring to us the continuing elimination of self deception, delusion, ignorance, superstition, the supernatural or obscure limiting beliefs especially in the face of adversity. Science helps us to release ourselves from foolish whims, dogma, fear or unsubstantiated flimsy fashionable beliefs of the multitudes. All these things influence, if not control our thinking, choices and decisions. Greater mastery of these life influencers gives us better mastery of ourselves.

Neuroscience helps us to understand all those things we take for granted or had not even noticed. It answers the question why we have senses like intuition and telepathic skills. Although no one has ever taught us what these are or how they work, they are in our constant use and important to our general success in life. Science, medical science and neuroscience enables us to focus with precision and recognise a better truth. But first we have to overcome one important hurdle.

THE TRUTH IS NOT FOR EVERYONE ONLY FOR THOSE WHO SEEK IT

From the earliest philosphers to the first and subsequent developments of modern psychology, mankind drew theoretical insights into what happened inside the brain and mind. Many were misguided indeed dangerous manipulating dogmas. One of the most limiting, which many people still belive to be true, is that it is dangerous to medle with the mind. However, medling with the mind to find what we are naturally good at or what thinking behaviours do not serve us well, is the begining of change and geater success in whatever we do with our lives. Take this to another level and it is how we may achieve the highest performance but notably free of stress. This type of meddling is based on observing the brain's natural behaviours and then modeling new thinking processes that achieve faster, better and higher performance with ease, even if that does include an above average degree of planning and effort.

At the age of twentyfour I realised I possessed a healing gift. Later in developing this gift I discovered the critical factor is in working with the mind in the way it likes to work at its best. The first principle of this was learning to accept it at face value and have no limiting beliefs about my healing ability.

Someone said, "Everything we are capable of thinking is possible." Although fundamentally true, this may be a bit of a stretch for many people. However looking back at history we come to understand that just about everything really is possible. The key to understanding this concept is in understanding how the mind works, especially the mechanics of achievement. This is precisely what I did to understand myself and how my model of alternative healing works. This is also how I helped the healing of my own burnout. It is how I developed and managed the next stage of creating a new way of life and a new future for myself that worked in unison and harmony with my inherent talents. This was when I realised burnout was actually an intelligence intent on preventing me from continuing to live the life that had so ably and brutally stopped me in my tracks.

"Know thyself" as a guidance to our greater achievement, is as valid today as ever it was for the ancient Greek philosophers. Then as now, paying attention to the multitudes or fashionable trends and their beliefs while ignoring what works well for ourselves; invariably results in regrettable folly.

Knowing ourselves focuses our attention on self leadership; it also develops intuitive skills. The more we do this the better our understanding of subconscious intelligence. Experience of ourselves and careful assessment of what we are told and what we believe, determines the outcome of our efforts and our lives. Using intuitive wisdom and the discipline of substantiated validation of everything in our lives may be a mouthful but it is as good as it gets when considering personal performance and achievement.

"Know thyself and thou shalt know all the mysteries of the gods and the universe," may be a stretch too far for most. Yet, "to know thyself first know thy mind," has a greater meaning most can hopefully recognise and do more than momentarily ponder thereupon.

Developing a healing gift certainly caused me to question my sense of identity. At the same time developing a career as an entrepreneur focused my attention on what I was capable of doing. So many changes in my life set up conflicts between who I had previously thought I was and what I had aspired to relative to the life I was living. Ignoring these disparities without changing or rationalising one side or the other; only leads to internal and emotional stress. Having an independent mind set, I did my best to ignore these conflicting notions of identity and function. Of course they steadily destabilised my inner balance and certainly my long standing hopes and dreams. Shutting out my internal mentor constantly working to get me to deal with these issues, was, I am sure an important part of my eventual burnout.

As with everyone else, pushing performance boundaries is not the problem. The real issue is the imbalance and stressors we create by the default limitations of our overall life style and thinking patterns. Whether for our own enterprise or as a company employee, pursuing a project, knowing what we want to achieve and passion for it, are vital to success. The dangerous trap for a workaholic such as myself is that passionate focus becomes tunnel vision and a succession of adrenalin bursts, which are highly addictive. The result of, which means we forget about not so apparent personal needs such as family, health, balance, friends, holidays, fun and happiness. Without respecting these things and properly managing passion, it all eventually turns into growing stressors and then overwhelming stress. Failure to deal with the stressors, our thinking becomes controlled by them and that causes more stress. How we react to our stressors determines how we manage change. Change only comes by self analysis, self leadership and pushing our limiting boundaries. Stressors limit development and progress because they feed limiting emotions into our thinking patterns and that is how we block our own progress. When limiting emotions take control of thinking; performance suffers. Dreams fade, become corrupted or get lost so they frequently die simply for the lack of continuing to believe in their meaning and purpose.

After more than twenty years of growing stress, I realised I was in trouble and needed to stop the world and get off for a rest or a complete change. I recognised being permanently exhausted but like many entrepreneurs, I drove myself on relentlessly. Unexpectedly, after a few more years of growing stress, I moved into a period of energetic activity and the tiredness vanished. I was once again rising to the greatest challenges and on a roll of adrenalin and enjoying it. I took every advantage of this feel good bonanza and it led to more activity and even less balance. This proved to be the frantic storm before the calm inactivity, silence and the numbness of a burnout crisis.

Oh yes, my world stopped still but this was not in my business or life plan. This sudden inactivity should have been a major anxiety for me because 98% of my thinking and performance activity had run into a wall of numbness. Old habits die hard as my first reaction was to keep going. That is when I found burnout is precisely what it says on the box. There is no "keep going," this is the train of my life jumping its tracks. Marooned and temporally incapable of helping myself, I was clearly going nowhere fast. My family doctor ordered me to take a vacation immediately. It was then that I found knowing myself proved to be the greatest support I had. I doubt it was my doctor's intention but for the first time that holiday gave me the space to begin analysing my life. It took a few days of lying on the beach, with nothing else to do before I understood why radical change was not simply important, it was vital and I really had no alternative option.

Burnout by its nature demands instant change. Slowly I discovered it was a holding stage for a healing process. This healing is the act of deciding what change is the best change. The healing was a critical period for self analysis and a new leadership. The first leadership is an internal intelligence called the 7th Sense Survival and Self Protection. Initially it sets up a "no go" mind process known as the "Want to but cannot syndrome." My first reactions were to try to get back to my life. That is when I recognised the power and control of my new 24/7 companion." Clearly it was not about to allow me to return to anything that in any way resembled my life before the burnout crisis; the biggest mistake of my life.

When I went through burnout, life coaching was in its infancy and the medical or neuroscience professions knew little about this growing problem of high stress burnout. Therefore, all I had was in knowing myself and my intuition to help me make the most of my predicament. I found the most fundamental aspect of analysing what I had become, was being able to refer back to what level of stress had appeared as normal and therefore mostly went unnoticed. This allowed me to determine what I needed to change in order to get me onto a new track. It is much the same as making any journey. Only by knowing where we are can we plan a route to what we want, where we want to go and how to get there. The difficulty with burnout is that if what we want is what we had before the burnout that is definitely no longer possible. Hence, we have, "the want to but cannot syndrome." This is because the innate survival and self protection intelligence is blocking the way back to more deadly burnout, namely "sudden death syndrome."

Confucius said, *"It is impossible to step into the same river twice,"* This is because the water is not only constantly moving forward; it is affected by turbulents, thus continually changing its shape and character. The message is that life and everything in it relentlessly moves forward. If we hope to succeed we have to be sure to persistently move forward with it and should we attempt to move forward into old and bad habits, we throw ourselves into the disharmony of fighting and blocking ourselves. In the extreme situation of burnout we need this iron hand to prevent any of our thinking that is still tied to and managed by the thinking behaviours, which got us into burnout. Apart from the medical issues involved, the psychological side of burnout seems to be designed to prevent us doing anything that is associated with what we did to get to burnout in the first place.

Being a dedicated and perpetual entrepreneur, when burnout struck the first abundantly clear aspect was the fact it was forcing me to run my life in a way completely contrary to all that came before. With nothing else to do, as soon as I was able, I began planning my future and that was naturally getting back to business. The burning question was, which parts had to change and how. The fact my father was dying when I was eight years old meant I did not have his guidance during the most critical stage of my life. The net result was a large gap in my understanding of myself and life, I recognised I was totally responsible for my plight. After burnout, going back to all that had marked my former thinking processes helped me to find the answer to a different thinking direction. I was aware of experiencing extreme limitations as to what I could think as the *"Want to but cannot syndrome"* familiar to all burnout victims, pulverised any creative thinking. What became apparent to me was how my internal survival intelligence systems were at that stage actually guiding my thinking patterns. This was like watching myself and my new thinking from a remote or meta position.

In hindsight I understand the frustration as my innate intelligence had taken over my life. Intuitively I sensed a future but not being allowed to know what it was. This is like being on a train that has stopped abruptly in the middle of nowhere. The frustration is always the same in the fact there is no information why the train has made an unscheduled stop or when the train is expected to continue forward on its journey.

As I began developing an acceptance of living with burnout, it had become obvious that knowing and aiming for what I wanted was out of the question. At this stage my subconscious survival and self protection intelligence ensured any creative thoughts I had for my future were on a very tight lead. At this stage I recognised the all important, "do not interfere" that had become so important to my support healing.

By other accounts and personal experience, burnout takes roughly four years to emerge from but this does not mean one is ever free from the experience. One wrong attempt to move backwards or prematurely forward is sufficient to activate once again the iron hand of the *"want to but cannot"* syndrome.

Moving forward out of burnout was itself a journey of discovery. I really did discover how this *"want to but cannot"* syndrome was intolerant of any interference on my part. Crossing that red line, meant I would be hit by a profound mental and physical fatigue, rendering me incapable of anything but sleeping.

Thereupon, I accepted that first I had to focus on allowing my innate healer to do the healing. I got the message that the less I interfered with my own ideas and the more I listened to intuitive guidance, the quicker progress I would make. This was a challenging situation for me but eventually, I accepted, only when I was ready would I be let into the secret of my own future. This actually proved itself to be true. When it came it was no sudden blinding inspirational insight. It turned out to be further developing my studies and the writing that I had intuitively started as a distraction of at least doing something creative to fill my days.

Anew part of this distraction was my interest and research into stress and burnout. I discovered the most common phenomenon about burnout is that it is like a volcano. With a little self awareness and openness to comments from family, friends and colleagues, the symptoms are clearly apparent. However, when it comes to the crisis proper, one never sees it coming until the moment it explodes into life. My burnout crisis was similar to a volcano. When a volcano blows its top and settles down, the landscape is changed forever. There is no immediate normal, it is something that has to evolve and getting it as right as possible is so important it cannot be left to our old thinking patterns. This is a good time to revisit psychometric test analysis and guidance also finding a mentor or life coaching support.

When burnout strikes we are changed forever. What may not be so apparent is the fact that our thinking behaviour and habits are forced to change. When a volcano lava flow or ash cloud crosses the countryside, ancient footpaths, roads, railways, homes, schools, factories and bridges are gone forever. Then the authorities are forced to build new services elsewhere home owners are forced to find another abode and workers forced to find different jobs or employers.

I was aware the only way forward for me to a new future was to trust my innate intelligence and be sure I did not interfere. Long before my own burnout I had been attracted to read two books written by people who had been through their own burnout. In the lead up to burnout I recognised the extreme stress but did not realise my personal volcano was about to blow. At that time I was on a high and pulling rabbits out of hats like never before. How could I imagine such a thing could happen to me? When it did, thanks to those books I understood exactly what had happened moments after the crisis struck. As the crisis peak subsided, I constantly asked the question "what now?" The only answer was to put my self-analysis to work to understand the prolonged high stress I imposed upon myself that had indefatigably changed my life for good.

One sign I had no idea as being significant, was that patients for healing had slowed to a trickle a month or two before the burnout crisis. Usually animals know there is a natural catastrophe about to happen and they leave a certain area. Perhaps by telepathy prospective patients intuitively knew there was something wrong. As the burnout crisis subsided I became more and more intrigued by how it came about and the many characteristics of its symptoms. I found myself fascinated by this new phenomenon in my life just as I had been working on understanding how my healing gift worked. Like the healing, I had made considerable progress to this end but with a basket of segmented understandings without the whole thing gelling into a complete process. As the months and years rolled by so many missing pieces were accounted for. As this change took place many parallels were observed in healing others as in my innate burnout healing. First was the evidence of important subconscious intelligence such as the "want to but cannot" syndrome and the clear strategies of the, "7th Sense Survival and Self Protection," intelligence. The former is self explanatory but the second showed itself to be far more complex with wide ranging elements.

After the burnout crisis there was clearly no question of me healing anyone until I had healed myself. This proved to be a classic case of achieving more by doing less. That may be understandable when considering the whirlwind life I had been living up to burnout. Albeit sudden, this passive stance allied with progressive analysis of my situation in a natural self coaching manner helped me to see new solutions. Subsequently it was burnout that pushed me into the study of neuroscience. Although this captured my interest, I had no idea it would help me out of that burnout mess or become so important to my way forward.

The *"want to but cannot"* syndrome had stopped any of my plans however it did not interfere with my study of how I got into burnout. The following years of studying stress and subconscious performance strategies and programs became a considerable part of my life. I had already discovered that one reason why subconscious high performance programs are so effective is because there is no conscious interference or stress in the subconscious mind. Just as I concluded this is important to support healing for others, it is hardly surprising it proved itself critical in healing my own burnout.

Unexpectedly, this process created a new paradigm of alternative therapy combining support healing, NLP, life coaching and neuroscience. The mind processes I had discovered in perfecting my own healing began to match up with those necessary for developing performance strategy programs for high performance without stress. This provoked many other important links between neuroscience and support healing. In short, they both highlighted what should be working but is not. This development led to a process of adapting natural mind patterns to learn how to get ahead of growing challenges and any subsequent stress. This developed into a process to gather existing stress and emotional stressors behind a virtual stress barrier where they can do no harm. Consequently these mind processes evolved into automatic, quick and practical ways to control stress and stressors rather than being controlled by them.

Further down the road of research this new alternative healing/neuroscience paradigm opened up the possibility of creating new subconscious thinking patterns and performance strategies. These are better suited to a fast changing world than the old far less performing ideas most of us use and well past their use by date. Retrospective analysis of my style of support healing and this new paradigm began to provide more answers as to how my support healing really worked.

For many years I had recognised myself in high stress and at times an overwhelming stress situation. I resorted to the same strategy as most soon to become burnout victims do. I drove myself and my determination to perform regardless. Convinced this demonstrated my strength of personal leadership and capability to manage my businesses, hindsight showed these strategies only led to more and higher stress. Progressive mistakes out of high stress thinking continually raised my stress by creating more mistakes. I found the recommended solutions designed to lower my stress actually raised it. The usual reason for this was due the frustrations in finding at best any benefits of sports, meditation, yoga, etc., were only slight and short lived. Getting to know myself after burnout showed how little at that time the stress therapists understood about emotional intelligence, and its importance in really effective stress therapy.

Getting to know myself paved the way to recognising the multitude of centres of intelligence within the body, brain and mind. Having read much about the innate healing intelligence, the immune intelligence and how intelligence is moved around the body by hormones and neurotransmitters, opened doors to thinking about myself in a different way. This paved the way to recognising the fact there are a multitude of centres of intelligence within the body for each organ, gland, intervening muscles, ligaments, nerves, veins, tissue, skin, indeed every cell within the body. Extensive study of these centres of intelligence showed me how they work and how they interact with emotional intelligence and thus how to work with or influence them in the best way possible. This led to understanding a new paradigm of the innate healer also further developing all I had learnt about my support healing.

At this level, knowing myself was becoming too complicated but with the aid of the new healing paradigm, I had found how to overcome this difficulty. It was just as Dr Deepak Chopra had said in his book Quantum Healing page 41. *"The frustrating reality as far as medical researchers are concerned, is that we already know that the living body is the best pharmacy ever devised. It produces diuretics, painkillers, tranquilizers, sleeping pills, antibiotics, and indeed everything manufactured by the drug companies, but it makes them much, much better. The dosage is always right and given on time; side effects are minimal or nonexistent; and the directions for using the drug are included in the drug itself, as part of its built in intelligence."* He also says; *"Our own inner intelligence is far superior to any we can substitute from the outside."* Furthermore; *"The body must be credited with an immense fund of know-how."*

As the evidence of how my support healing gift unravelled, four things became abundantly clear. 1. The body must be credited with an immense fund of know-how intelligence. 2. That intelligence is superior to anything I might consider as helpful, therefore; 3. Support the patient's body to do its own healing and 4. Do not interfere.

This stage it so obvious; to succeed, I did not need to gain a multiple doctorate in the unimaginable intelligence that makes me or my patient's tick. The key was in knowing all my brain/mind/body centres of intelligence were their own oracle. These centres of intelligence know everything there is to know about me so why reinvent this particular wheel of knowledge. Why keep a dog and bark myself? To improve and refine my support healing, all I had to do was learn how to communicate with this intelligence.

It quickly became clear that telepathy was the only viable solution to how to communicate with my own or the patient's subconscious mind. The next question to appear was how was I to know that I had done that successfully. Of course the results spoke for themselves. However, there was another answer that had been within earshot from the beginning. It was just a matter of spotting that it always occurred when a healing was successful. What it was and how it seemed it could be so easily missed was a significant step forward. I had always noted the sign; I just did not take any notice only because I had not known what it represented.

Therefore, the success of my alternative healing was in knowing where the best information is held and definitely not interfering with what I might perceive to be helpful. With the guidance of my growing studies of neuroscience I began to recognise, understand and prosper anew by direct support of my emotional intelligence, explicit creative intelligence, intuitive intelligence, telepathic intelligence, subconscious ambition intelligence, 7th sense of survival and self protection intelligence, implicit intelligence also as many other subconscious centres of intelligence just waiting to be put to work.

Perhaps this may be summed up as a perfect example of applying what Albert Einstein said, *"Any idiot can know but understanding is what really makes the difference."*

The point here is there is no limit or end to the process of learning and understanding, the key to real success is to understand how best to learn. So in this vein this book "Will the Real Healer Please Stand Up" the upgrade to Activating Spontaneous Healing published in 2007, does its best to extend a greater understanding in order to eliminate ignorance, superstition and the supernatural by better understanding ourselves. This is particularly as far as understanding the power of inner healing intelligence and therefore caring for our health, happiness, and especially our emotional and feelings intelligence.

When I discovered I possessed a gift of healing it was evident I could simply put my hands on a sick person and they would quickly recover. Whatever I did was 100% intuitive because at that stage I had no structured training of how to use the gift. Not understanding the principles of my healing gift proved to be temporary. This was due to a spiritual healer and a leader of a spiritual church who got to hear about my healing coming to see me. These two insisted on taking me in hand and making sure I followed a strict spiritual dogma. I was surprised to find this had the effect of considerably diminishing my healing capability. Nonetheless, this turn of events drove a greater need to understand how my healing gift worked. I needed to understand why my healing potential had changed with the intervention of my self-appointed spiritual healer/mentors. I was certain it was not just a case of going back to what I did before. It was important for me to understand how my healing worked and why the spiritual practices I had been advised to follow were so damaging. Eventually I found the spiritual healing was essentially handed down dogma and mostly a game of Chinese whispers, fogged by smoky mirrors and ego driven interference dressed up as good intentions.

In my capacity as a support healer, I quickly discovered I was the last resort for my patients. This was after exhausting all other medical solutions. My patients would usually recount the treatment horrors they had been through to no avail. Despite this, I asked them to accept that medical science, our hospitals, doctors and nurses are quite incredible in what they can do. They always have to be our first port for all health issues. This proved to be of some value because it led my patients to become interested in why treatments that had worked for many others had not worked for them. Later on I will explain why this is so important and how this understanding leads to releasing who the real healer is and how to support it to do its job without interfering.

DEDICATIONS

I dedicate this book to all those people who came to me for healing. First, they were directly instrumental in aiding me to fully understand how and why their healing worked.

They made this book possible due to their trust and confidence in me even though they had never met me before. I found it fascinating they could believe in something steeped in myth and in general still remains so. It was through each encounter that I learnt so much about myself and my gift. Both successes also the apparent failures were equally important to understand how a so called healing gift really worked. This understanding led to how to work with it in the very best way so it could be at its most potent.

Like a fine sword, it is only when tempered and tested in the white heat of the blacksmiths fire and imperfections are beaten out on his anvil that it may eventually rise to all challenges placed upon it. In this testing of my healing gift I came to realise that everyone has the potential of healing another to a considerable degree though they may not know it. One thing I remain constantly aware of is the fact that my healing experience is unique as is that of all healers whether orthodox or alternative. The difference in my case, is the less I tried to be the healer the better the healing worked.

I also acknowledge my parents and all my ancestors whose genetic programmes, beliefs, values, fears, traumas, joys, ambitions and love, trickled down the generations of genetic programming to create this gift and who I am today. With no idea of the genetic programs they were responsible for modifying and passing down the genetic line, each has participated in writing this book.

Robert P. Denton

A MESSAGE FROM THE AUTHOR

Every day medical science recognises a little more about our internal or innate healing and body management and their remarkable intelligence systems. That knowledge is to some degree wrapped in jargon better understood to the medical professions. One purpose of this book is to move aside at least part of this veil hiding some facts we can all understand and incorporate in our better daily management of ourselves. Experiential healing examples illustrate that when alternative healing is exercised free of the healers well meaning interference, it is able to help in many cases where orthodox medicine alone sets itself up to fail. This is not suggesting that the majority of orthodox medical treatment is wrong, more the case it misses unique needs of specific people particularly their emotional intelligence and their inner healer. As stated above Dr. Chopra highlights many reasons why this can be the case. In addition I discovered the importance of emotional intelligence and why subconscious emotional trauma needs to be healed before medical treatment could be effective.

The question is then; why doesn't our innate healing system intelligence work perfectly so we never get sick? Although emotional intelligence is involved, the whole answer to this question is still a mystery to medical researchers. Apart from minor to serious accidents and transmittable diseases, it is clear that genetic errors in DNA programming are the cause of many medical problems. Some of these are active from birth and others are triggered by life, toxic substance and traumas to the system. The possibilities seem to be endless as apparently minor issues to one can be quite different and devastating to others

Any conditions affecting physical health are manifest by varying degrees of discomfort, pain and disability. All being well, they are treatable via our internal pharmacy. If this cannot rise to the occasion then we need the external support of doctors, hospitals, surgeons and the high street pharmacies we are more familiar with. If these services do not do the trick then it is likely something like emotional trauma is blocking healing from somewhere deep inside the patient's mind.

This leads us to emotional injuries which are another major cause of both minor and major health issues, also why both internal and external medications are powerless. This is why support healing, NLP therapy, life coaching, transgenerational therapy and support healing can make the difference. I include case history examples in the following text and specific case history chapters that demonstrate emotional power.

There is a great deal of talk about emotional intelligence but how many people truly understand what it is, how it comes about, also why particularly emotional trauma can be such a powerful obstacle. I would describe emotional intelligence starting with why it is so powerful. Why and how does it literally control what happens within our bodies and how and why it is so adept at controlling our decisions, choices and behaviours? In a nut shell, our physical bodies are made of matter and for that matter to take any shape or purpose it has to have energy. That energy has to have information to guide its form to take the ideal shape, structure and purpose. For purpose to have direction and performance it has to have beliefs and values (programs of performance) in order that it may perform appropriately.

That is not the end. Each cell has its life cycle, its senescence or aging program also its apoptosis or programmed cell death. It has its objectives and performance. All this comes under the general heading of cell or DNA programming. For it to achieve its goals it has to have a sense of identity and that means it has emotional control. Emotional intelligence is essentially that which monitors, checks and balances each cell's internal state and interaction with all other cells. Yes, all fifty billion of them. In the simplest terms it can be said that each body cell has its own emotional identity and thus a programmed purpose.

If we take a quantum leap to analyse our thinking, functioning bodies, we realise why just like all cells, our minds or more precisely our thinking processes also require the guidance of beliefs, values, identity and purpose. These are necessary so we can function successfully in achieving our dreams, goals, daily needs, obligations and tasks, many of, which we have little idea are like puppet masters within our gene programming. Beliefs and values are the highway rules, codes and laws, which keep our unique thinking on track whether they are right, wrong, good or bad.

When the physical body is injured in any way we experience discomfort and pain. These signals come from cell guiding intelligence. Emotions come into the picture as internal signals alerting their support systems into action when beliefs, values, identity and purpose are under attack or injured. If we physically injure ourselves, we will most likely suffer a proportional pain response, which says, "do not do that to yourself again." If someone flatters or attacks our beliefs, values, identity or purpose and performance, we may experience varying degrees of response from joy to emotional embarrassment to anger and outward aggression.

The reason the beliefs and values we use consciously and subconsciously are so powerful, is because coming from our subconscious intelligence they appear instantly. Harmony of this wide ranging process is what may be described as balanced emotional intelligence. This may be further indicated as being in a state where every cell and thought in the body and mind is in perfect harmony and communication with all other cells. That is to say in a perfect state of mental and body health. This also includes a complete synergy with the surrounding environment. Some believe this extends to the limits of the universe and beyond. This may seem impossible to achieve because it is as close as we can get to the spark of life and the source of all energy. Nonetheless, it is powerful because it has the intelligence, (Einstein's soup of energy and information) which means it is driven by the spark of life. Emotional intelligence is powerful because it is essentially the driving force and cybernetic pilot that gives direction to life itself.

We all have a purpose program within our DNA programming, which I describe as "subconscious ambition." Subconscious ambition may be influenced and to some degree managed by emotional intelligence. This is why we each have beliefs and values, it is when our conscious beliefs and values exceed the parameters of our emotional intelligence beliefs that we find ourselves blocked and unable to be or perform as normal. This is the basis of the "want to but cannot" syndrome. When I pushed my capability and performance to such limits, I was sabotaging my emotional intelligence to such a degree; I drove my stress levels up through the roof. This meant my body flooded with cortisol to such an extent that my spark of life was in mortal danger. When I pushed the limits of my emotional intelligence, it first shut me down by throwing a gigantic spanner in the works and then applied the "want to but cannot" syndrome, leaving me incapable of doing myself more damage and that is what I understand burnout is.

When we have a physical injury the controlling beliefs and values of harmony are screaming foul, thus we have an intellectual emotionally driven physical pain pointing to where the injury is. The burning message of the moment is to do something before the pain gets even worse.

When our controlling beliefs and values that keep our sense of balance, worth, identity and purpose are injured we are likely to experience emotional kickback. For example; by harsh or cruel things other people do or say to us or we allow ourselves to be pushed into stamping on our own fundamental beliefs and values; sooner or later we will revolt. This is due to the troubling circumstances causing emotional intellectual distortions and confusion and these manifest themselves in various and many forms of emotional also psychosomatic pain. Our emotional intelligence is trying to rebalance conscious purpose and performance with subconscious programmed purpose and performance. Because this process originates from our veritable core, we are usually aware of even the slightest emotional change. Our problems start when we take no notice of this intelligence. Taken to their extremes, they become emotional traumas and their consequences can be; in the worst circumstances; catastrophic to our emotional and mental state and therefore also to body, mind and physical health.

Upset this balance sufficiently to cause confusion and pain and we see why we are capable of behaving in unusual and self limiting or ultimately self destructive ways. This is almost certainly why power corrupts. As I learnt to push all sorts of performance boundaries in the pursuit of my career and objectives, I sensed this power by the constant release of adrenalin as a reward for achieving. Although I was not consciously aware of what I was doing, I became addicted to it so I pushed myself and my beliefs and values to extremes to keep the adrenalin highs coming.

By purposefully changing our beliefs and values, we can improve our performance and then we activate a rather unusual emotional intelligence, which signals we have "done good." Then we may experience different emotions of relief, extreme happiness, joy and ecstasy. This is when we are rewarded with copious quantities of a cocktail of feel good endorphins, serotonin, dopamine and adrenalin rushing around our blood stream so that every cell in our body can enjoy this elixir of life and join in the celebration. Frequently this manifests itself in emotional tears of joy. When experiencing this feel-good cocktail it is so addictive it corrupts our beliefs and values so that we can keep pushing the boundaries of performance. Perhaps that is why we have the counter strategy of anti-climax to get our feet back on the ground. This addiction can be anything from pushing ourselves to extremes by breaking all the rules of a balanced life as I did, also to financial corruption in companies or corruption by breaking all the rules of honest business. This also affects governmental leadership in self aggrandisement and theft of a countries wealth.

The toughest, hardest, thickest skinned people are all susceptible to their emotional intelligence and emotional release. This is the reason why NLP therapists and life coaches and indeed my own support healing are careful to have a box of paper tissues in easy reach of their clients or patients. When the coaching or support healing helps the patient to break through any limiting emotional blockages, this is when the inner feel-good hormones and neurotransmitters release the "well done - good job" feeling and then but not always, the tears of emotional relief break out. The reason for this is conscious and subconscious intelligence beliefs and values being re-harmonised. This may mean moving forward or updating beliefs and values that got stuck in the past. The effect of this harmonisation is to make a quantum leap forward to where we should be in relation to our fundamental purpose.

What began to make some sense is that the problem with orthodox medical treatment that fails to perform in one patient when it is known to have been effective in previous patients, is that if the treatment ignores the fundamental emotional reason for or linked to the illness then it blocks itself. The patient is then fighting against its own superior emotional intelligence so powerfully it is capable of blocking any treatment.

Patients coming to me were predominately concerned with cancers of varying types for, which medical treatment had failed and their doctor's prognosis was not good. In some cases the doctor's advice was go and see a healer, try whatever you can. In the following chapters I aim to explain why this was certainly the case for those people who asked for my help. Other conditions ranged from healing anything from painful eye conditions, to profound mental blockages, to severed nerves, to a boy unstoppably slipping into a coma because his body was no longer responding to dialysis treatment. From a simple observation of the range of conditions presented to me, my only conclusion is that it can only be the patient's innate healing intelligence aided by the release of emotional blockages that could affect so many complex healings and at an incredible speed.

Here I express my thoughts, feelings, experiences, findings and research of fifty years working in this field. I have taken note of many eminent writers, medical doctors, neuroscientists and researchers some of which are listed within the bibliography. This is to illustrate a better and clearer understanding of the body/brain innate healing systems intelligence, also why my support healing led to so many cases of successful spontaneous healing.

In this book I explain the story about something I was practicing over more than three decades that helped countless people. The case histories over those years are remarkable. Therefore, please read this book with an open mind, though what you will read may seem unbelievable or go against some or even many of your established beliefs and values.

As with all research, today in June 2017 after an interval of ten years since the original book, many new discoveries medical, neuroscience and within my own support healing research have widened the scope, knowledge and understanding of the intricacies of activating spontaneous healing. In those intervening years both medical and neuroscience have helped me to extend and further develop my earlier discoveries and theories of an alternative way of working with the body's innate healing systems and with their incredible intelligence.

One of the most dynamic areas of my research has been the growing understanding of the innate healing system centres of intelligence. These are layers of intelligence beyond each of the billions of cells that make up the human body. They contain their own specific intelligence. Glibly, we talk of DNA programming as if it is done and dusted. This combined programming of intelligence is required to form all the parts of the body plus how to manage them in relation to all other parts. This is the intelligence that sustains the spark of life. The intelligence of every cell determines how each part functions, which determines its level of performance, which in turn determines our state of health and personal performance at any given time. When any of those cells lose their management intelligence is when things begin to go wrong. Centres of intelligence cannot fall prey to health conditions like cancer but they have their own dangers and susceptibilities mostly in the form of blocking emotional traumas. These are higher levels of intelligence and they determine those traumas must be healed before anything else. They also control precisely what is acceptable in terms of external support healing whether that is orthodox medical or alternative therapy.

One patient had difficulty to fully enjoy and excel at his favourite sports of cricket and tennis. This proved to be because of just one muscle in his right eye underperforming. This defective intelligence and performance caused the focus of the eye to flick or jump when an incoming cricket or tennis ball was precisely eight feet away from him. At this crucial moment he lost sight of the ball for a split second. Given that a cricket ball may travel at any speed up to approximately 161 km/h and a tennis ball, 263km/h, a split second is long enough to cause havoc in his capability and performance, resulting in a poor return strike on the ball or missing it altogether.

Only in recent years have scientists been able to understand DNA coding and point out inherited genetic faults. Without that science, this patient's ophthalmic specialist was still able to witness and pinpoint the errant muscle but he could do little other then recommend eye exercises. The probable reason why support healing worked in this case was not revealed for another thirty years. The answers emerged as research on exoskeletal support for spinal cord injuries was publicised in 2016. More on this new research is explained further on. The essential element is the exoskeletal support enables the brain to bypass the damaged spine to regain control of the lower limbs and other functions. There was no physical exoskeleton for this man's eye. Nonetheless, it appears this healing case had enabled the patient's eye management intelligence to reprogram his other eye muscles to behave as an exoskeleton would. Thus so; the one faulty eye muscle may not have been changed but it was no longer capable of causing further limitations of critical high performance eye movement.

Today this is not so surprising as it is now possible to write and install new behaviour programs for high performance strategy creation without upsetting basic subconscious beliefs, values or emotional intelligence. This mind, body/mind process takes a matter of hours not days or months. This is possibly just as it is feasible to upgrade a computer program that is not performing as well as expected. The above case demonstrates how just one very small muscle or belief can spoil performance, undermine effort, break concentration also unnecessarily raise stress levels.

The most common of all causes able to be identified were various forms of emotional blockages. Many patients were consciously aware of these and accepted their long term presence without considering any form of treatment was necessary. First they did not consider themselves as needing any sort of psychological therapy and second they considered it all part of life and did not realise emotional issues could upset their health and work performance. They acknowledged emotional scars had marred their life and happiness to some degree but never to the extent of realising they could lead to a cancer tumour. A further issue was how they could identify a sense of being emotionally off balance from the time of a trauma but gradually they became used to it and pushed it away so at worst it seemed to only bother them occasionally. What they did not realise was that it was working in their subconscious intelligence 24/7.

During the past twenty years the positive and negative effects of emotional intelligence on our performance have been recognised far better. When the emotional intelligence is positive our performance potential is practically unlimited. When the emotional intelligence is traumatised, it is invariably sufficiently disturbed so it becomes out of balance. Untreated that has long term consequences to our homeostasis (general well-being) and thus to overall performance.

Nature relentlessly continues to evolve in the pursuit of perfection to match the prevailing environment. Unfortunately for us; the speed of our changing societies and environments, have far outpaced our natural or willing evolution to stay abreast of modern demands. This means keeping and developing what we have becomes daily more difficult. This is particularly apparent as we get past our prime in our mid thirties. As this process is now understood so much better, it is becoming obvious our prime is much younger than most would prefer to believe. Some may be high performs into their seventies but it takes longer and more stressful. Therefore, to stack the dice in our own favour for a longer stretch of high performance, we are wise to constantly know ourselves and work at keeping our beliefs, values, identity and purpose up to date with our permanently changing personal, work and social environment.

Given the level of trials, tribulations, hereditary diseases and imperfections, it is clear there is much evolving to come just to maintain a status quo. The mind, body, body-mind and its centres of intelligence at any moment are the current state of each beings evolution. Feelings, emotions, intuition, centres of innate intelligence and conscious thinking are states of being, relative to specific moments, in a constant state of change. These combined states of intelligence can be either our greatest friend or worst enemy to homeostasis. That is all wrapped up in one perpetually changing package of beliefs, values, behaviours, habits conscious and subconscious thinking patterns. Mostly all this goes unnoticed or completely ignored whenever our awareness signals a problem.

Our one massive saving grace is that our combined innate intelligence holds all information about us. Therefore, it is also the only intelligence to understand what is good. When the system brakes-down it knows what has gone wrong and precisely what is needed to fix it. This intelligence knows exactly what it can do itself also; what outside support it needs, in addition to what form and how it will accept it. The fly in the ointment is that we have not yet learnt all there is to know in how to help and care for ourselves.

This is precisely what I mean when I referred to medical science inadvertently setting itself up to fail. Given the right support our innate healing intelligence will respond quickly and easily to treatment. Even given the right medical treatment but no emotional support, wrong emotional support or interfering support, any form of treatment may fail. Where the treatment ignores the emotional aspects, the innate healing and emotional centres of intelligence are capable of self defeating acts by blocking any external help no matter how appropriate and well meaning.

Emotional intelligence is tied to our hopes, dreams, aspirations, goals, beliefs, values, behaviours and thus ultimate performance physically, consciously and subconsciously. Like everything in this natural world of evolution, each set of behaviours has its use by date and this is where many of our illnesses or life's problems originate. This is to say, of all those qualities listed above each fits into one of two categories of being 1. Valid and Supporting in the moment, or 2. Redundant and Disabling.

When we get stuck in redundant ways, emotional intelligence does its best to point out our errors. This is great except for the fact we do not understand this language and therefore mostly ignore the messages emotional intelligence sends us. It then reverts to sending us messages we cannot ignore because they are sufficiently painful and self limiting; these are referred to as psychosomatic conditions. Eventually we do something about blotting out the pain but ignore the emotional cause and thus we pay the price for buried emotions by thinking we know what we are doing. In a few words, these ignored or buried emotions are the imperceptible things that stifle or block emotional growth, creativity and success. Indeed also the body's immune and self healing systems and thus our general wellbeing.

Above all, what has changed in modern neuroscience in recent years continues to give me confidence in my conclusions as to how and why my support healing had been so successful. So many of my own observations and discoveries about activating spontaneous healing, are recognised or used in the field of orthodox medicine in various forms albeit in some cases unknowingly. Even if this is only recognised at the fringes of orthodox medical healing, this confidence is important for the reason it helps the process of healing to further evolve. Thus in knowing this part of myself, I directly demonstrate how and why I am mindful to always search for new understanding beyond the boundaries of assumed limits. The trick to continued success is therefore, not to be persuaded or blocked by negative, misinformation, limiting and outdated, redundant opinions. Keep on pushing the envelope of knowledge, change and performance but always with a careful eye on life balance supported by appropriately evolving beliefs, values and behaviours in compliance with one's environment and fundamental emotional intelligence parameters.

One part of my professional day job, was as a legal expert-witness. The world's legal profession rely heavily on established presidents (reliable beliefs and values held to be more or less universally true). When it comes down to specialised knowledge this is the minimum expert-witnesses are required to provide. That is fine but for the problem that those presidents tend to become overworked and thus corrupted to fit all manner of situations. Where expert witnesses have the capability to push the boundaries of knowledge, I found established presidents can become seriously lacking. This is largely due to changing circumstances governed by social, economical, science or engineering or professional developments. This brings me right back to the ancient Greek philosopher's warnings not to be persuaded by the masses. Before burnout, the key to my many legal case successes was related to knowing myself, also the depth of personal experience and my capability to make verifiable connections with less obvious associated issues. This capability had evolved due to my own efforts of persistently pushing the boundaries of my expertise by open minded detailed observation. This invariably gave fresh light and powerful arguments in the process of exposing the opposition's limitations and unravelling the underlying relevant facts, thus could give considerable bearing to the appropriate legal and just outcome.

In the same manner, knowing myself and my capacity to observe the fine detail, I was able to learn quickly from each new healing experience. This proved itself important to the success of developing my healing gift. That same attention to detail, especially to what is happening behind the scenes was important in the analysis of each healing case history. This gave me a broad basis from which to further grow; consequently affording a better support to my patients albeit without interfering.

Within the following chapters you will find how we as humans are so capable of hindering, stifling or even blocking our health and general success in life. Worst still, we do all that while thinking we do know what we are doing is right. That is without being aware of the full facts or the true meaning of those facts. This is the point I made earlier about the importance of knowing myself. This is in not interfering with what I think is right but using that knowledge and experience to develop my support healing by supporting the real subconscious intelligence that does know precisely what is right.

Before the burnout I thought I was doing all the right things for success in my businesses. It all proved to be smoke, mirrors and temporary success for my companies as they all turned to dust when burnout struck. In addition, this was certainly not success for my personal quality of life. The main problem was one of balance. This is to say my professionally dominated tunnel vision had excluded the person, blocked the balanced nurturing of my spark of life and my reason to be; all of which were important in creating those continual successes. This meant I was living by cannibalising my emotional intelligence until close to the point of there being nothing left to give.

Today the growing problem of complete imbalance and thus burnout, expands in tandem with the growing demands on highly capable and sensitive professional people. The risks are enormous. One European figure and now leader of an influential world body, who understands this, was asked if she would stand for president of France. She replied; *"Do you think I am crazy, whatever I do in life, I wish to retain my sanity."*

Clearly without caring correctly for the machinery that creates the successes, both those successes and the machinery are likely to sooner or later grind to a standstill as the entire process breaks down. This is what burnout is but it goes further because it triggers something else, which is far more devastating. The actual burnout crisis, in one foul swoop destroys all confidence and thus blocks all levels of performance. After the burnout crisis had begun to subside, the only thing I was able to do was to take the time to inspect myself. This was to assess how out of balance my life was and the real state of my physical and emotional health.

It became clear that in order to heal myself, I had to make many changes in my life style. Having identified where I had gone so wrong in my thinking, I was able to pin-point what I had inadvertently been doing with my life. Burnout included all the warning signs of what not to do in the future. This seemed to be so I would avoid making the same mistakes again that got me into burnout in the first place. It was this process that taught me how to go about healing myself without interfering in the process.

Hippocrates, born around 460 BC and regarded as the father of modern medicine, said to all emerging doctors, *"whatever you do, do no harm."*

The spiritualist dogma offered to me in the early days felt bizarre, therefore I sensed it was somehow intrusive and therefore at risk at the very least of some sort of deception and certainly if not hurtful it was unhelpful. My own discovery of not interfering is I believe roughly what Hippocrates meant by, *"do no harm."* This has been to always work with this inner intelligence and never interfere by ignoring it, working against it or indeed despite it.

I have noted how many spiritual and faith healers make a point of diagnosing their patient's problems. I am certain that alternative healing should never be a case of diagnosis, i.e. identifying causes. Even if those seem to be patently clear, at the least this is the work of the medical profession. From an emotional aspect, at its best or worst it will be hopelessly wrong because there is no knowing the innermost secret workings of any one conscious and subconscious mind. If the medical profession can get diagnosis wrong given all their resources, what chance does a healer have to get it right.

The important point for the alternative support healer is there is no benefit in them trying to understand the problems and the causes. This is because that amount of information would certainly lead to information-overwhelm. What is worse this would lead to their getting it all wrong resulting in pointless interference. Thereby, their interference will distract them from what they really can do that may be of some benefit to their patients.

In the case of emotional issues, I am convinced these are far better served by life coaching skills than trying some contrived alternative healing process. Life coaching has specific tried and tested skills to identify to ourselves what is not working in our thinking, our performance, our health or our lives and why.

Self coaching was only possible for myself by virtue of my own emerging need for brutal honesty. This is how I asked myself the questions that released the answers that led to the questions I was incapable of even considering let alone asking myself before the burnout. The positive outcome in doing this is that I began to support a better health balance of my own mind and body. The principle reason for this was for the first time I was encouraging underlying emotional issues to show themselves.

In the beginning of developing my healing gift, I was obliged to accept the generalised labels of spiritual or faith healer. I disliked both of these terms because I, like so many other people have no firm idea what those words really are supposed to represent. Researching this subject, I found faith and spirituality apparently have multiplicities of differing meanings to each one of us. This meant that faith or spiritual healing would certainly in my own case represent misguided assumptions, misconceptions for all that I was doing my best to understand. This was especially as intuitively in those early days, I felt that I was not the healer. I now will endeavour to explain this anomaly as I unravel what I believe my healing gift is all about.

Taught I was the healer and held the power of healing seemed to be evident as I was involved in some amazing healings notably cancers after medical treatment had failed. However, despite the repeated spiritual dogma I had a growing distaste there could be such a thing as spiritually induced healing wrapped up in mysterious quackery for which there was no confirmable evidence of what it was - that it actually worked or how it worked. Eventually, much to my pleasure, I understood how true this feeling proved to be. Whatever that was, I was certainly not the real healer and therefore had no intention of playing the role of doctor, surgeon or God's spiritual representative.

As I began to learn about the body's innate healing systems and their formidable intelligence, it became apparent I was somehow supporting the patient to kick start their own innate healing system into action. In later chapters I believe this becomes self explanatory but I will endeavour to explain how and why I came to this conclusion.

I had found trusting and following intuition and consciously doing very little else, proved preferable to following a contrived procedure of so called freeing stagnant energy in the patient. This may have its merits as that is essentially what a trained and licensed acupuncturist does. The ridiculousness of a healer achieving this with a few hours training or no training at all is evident when considering a qualified acupuncturist takes many years and possibly an entire life time to learn precisely how to do this effectively. As the myth and superstition had been replaced with rational understanding based on neuroscience and medical science, my support healing turned into a practical, explainable therapy. The first thing this clearly identified was how the body and indeed its inbuilt intelligence is its own greatest healer and pity anyone unqualified who has delusions of interfering.

Like any other gifted person, my particular gift of healing had to be developed in the right way to get the most out of it. Discovering it was essentially no different than a gifted musician, actor, writer, etc., further debunked any idea of undying faith or mystical and spiritual involvement. However, I did accept part of this gifted talent is a heightened intuitive and telepathic awareness. Not everyone is so familiar with these senses, which I do understand can so easily be misconstrued as spiritual intervention.

As my reputation grew it became apparent that more patients were suffering with cancer of one sort or another. Initially I just did what worked, which I will explain in due course. As time progressed and as some patients did not respond to the healing as well as others with the same condition, I was drawn to understanding why. This was not so I could interfere or bolster my ego; rather it was that I might find if I had previously inadvertently interfered in some way.

I began looking at the behaviour of cells, what controls them and how and why some cells go rogue. What became clear was how the body really is its greatest healer driven by an incomprehensibly capable innate healing intelligence. As you will note throughout this book, this intelligence has tremendous resources to constantly heal and keep itself in balance. The down side is that it also has the capability to be oblivious of alien organisms in its system and thus actively aid its own downfall. Evidence of this is seen in Aids, cancers, Alzheimer's and other rapid degenerative disease capable of fooling the immune system and "T" cells whose job it is to detect any interlopers. The fly in the ointment is how this intelligence can cause the innate healing systems to attack and destroy its own spark of life by apparently believing it is doing the right thing.

While evolved mind management programs have the capability to preserve a reasonably balanced state of health, the question was what had the power to upset such amazing intelligence. What has the power to block the very system its innate healing intelligence had evolved to protect itself and its beliefs, values, identity and purpose?

It is clear that radiation is a major danger. Toxic chemicals are known to be hazardous to our health. Chemicals apparently benign in the case of low doses are all capable of cell damage because by a drip, drip process they damage the DNA information and intelligence intended to keep the cells stable. When none of these elements are involved what else can cause such havoc to cell programming and stability? My observations suggest that in the case of each of my patients, there had been a marked emotional trauma or an enduring secret emotional fear at some stage in their life, which had been ignored or sometime literally buried alive in the furthest depths of their mind. Secondly, the fact their cancers were throwing their emotional balance into chaos every waking and sleeping minute as they faced the reality of their medical treatment having failed, indeed also the trauma of their premature death.

Within the orthodox medical profession it is well understood that emotional chaos such as living with a long term fear and trauma may cause the manifestation of physical conditions known as psychosomatic illnesses. My case histories indicated that if there is a powerful and deep set emotional blockage involved, which is not resolved as part of any orthodox treatment, then conventional medicine or surgery may fail to heal the condition. This failure at least led some people to ask me for my help albeit that it was as a last resort and packaged in the sentiment; why not, they had nothing to lose.

I believe the reason why my intervention made the difference was that it first supported the patient in healing their emotional blockage. There is more about this later. Once complete, their innate healing system was then able to heal themselves of their physical ailment. This apparent fact is notable in practically all cases. Particularly, in respect of the case histories of "Mark the racing car driver" and "Quarry workers" albeit neither involved cancer, the emotional elements were significant. Also this point underlines the uncommon case of Telepathy with a Rock, albeit this case had the right outcome, it was via quite an unusual process.

The conclusion is that if the critical emotional element is not addressed properly at the same time as orthodox medical treatment, then the body's internal intelligence seems to have the power to block both external treatments; also its own innate healing system. This paradoxical process appears to be the 7th Sense Survival and Self Protection Intelligence. This is to say, the same intelligence that initially blocked my recovery from burnout. Another paradox is the survival intelligence was right in doing its job as intended. This is by bringing my attention to the underlying beliefs, values, identity, purpose distortions, which led to overwork and forcing myself through high stress when I really did need a break. Thus, life balance and therefore; connected emotional issues became apparent as the principal cause of my health condition. My burnout was all the evidence I needed to understand that if limiting stress and emotional issues are allowed to persist, the potential knock-on effect may be significant.

By virtue of excessively focusing on the problem, it has the effect of accentuating it. Since these are emotional issues, the more they grow the more powerful they become. As the problem space becomes too dominant and stressful, there is little if any space for the solution to show itself. Therefore, if the solution to the emotion is well and truly stuck and cannot be released, it turns its energy inwards in a very bad way. This is the stage where an emotional stress turns into a physical reaction. It impacts on respective glands, which release hormones and neurotransmitters that cause psychosomatic conditions to manifest as real health issues.

Some of the complications appear to be aggravated by the fact internal intelligence systems are in it for the long haul and our conscious minds with what we think is right, simply gets in the way as we strive for short term and quick solutions.

When we focus all our attention on a problem to the degree it becomes dominant and therefore stressful, it may then morph into emotional frustrations, possibly anger and perhaps a feeling of being powerless. If then we become consumed by fear of what might happen next that can activate more production of the mind changing and stress hormone cortisol. When this happens whatever decisions we make they are likely to be the wrong ones, which naturally further aggravate the problem. At this late stage we become all consumed by the problem and thus we cannot see the forest for the trees, in which case we have even less chance of finding the solution.

The result is the perceived problem and underlying emotional trauma recycling around itself, thus eventually giving the impression it is bigger than it really is. By this stage we begin to feel there is no solution. That is when we may become demoralised or depressed. So what do we do, we continue with more of the same bad habits. At this point the negative emotional intelligence takes control. This is how we end up in a situation of the emotional tail of stress wagging the dog of confusion, frustration and poor performance, wellbeing, etc. This ultimately results in a life style of general disillusionment and possibly a further compounding stressful feeling of being lost.

Life coaching in all its forms came about because our lives have become dominated by ever more complex problems. Boil it down to its basics; life coaching is a highly focused compilation of natural success mind strategies. Life coaching is all to do with exposing well guarded conscious and subconscious limiting perceptions. In the worst cases unaided; these give power to limiting emotional traumas by keeping them from being observed, analysed and debunked as imposters or aliens in the system.

There are many coaching strategies designed to move the coachee's or client's thinking from the problem to their own workable and achievable solution. Consequently the undeniable fact is that life coaching is a powerful form of healing.

My support healing methods demonstrate other qualities including a heightened telepathic capability. However this works, it is similar to life coaching because it focuses on passive respect of psychological and therefore emotional intelligence and thus it consequentially avoids the risks of unhelpful interference.

Medical science already fully understands that untreated emotional traumas can lead to the appearance of associated psychosomatic, physical and psychological conditions. This is why psychotherapists already practice trauma therapy and specialist life coaches use coaching skills to affect the equivalent intended results but very likely in a fraction of the time. This is because life coaching works at the level of emotional intelligence and how the subconscious mind likes to work, not on the basis the mind is sick or broken.

The fundamental importance is for the therapist of whatever genre to avoid any belief they can possibly understand what lies behind any one health condition. The reason life coaching and my support healing work so quickly is almost certainly due to outwardly avoiding any interference. The toxicity of the most popular cancer treatment may be exceptionally bad because the treatment is forcing the innate healing systems and its internal intelligence centres to focus all their effort in fighting for their own survival. This may conceivably be one of many reasons why in certain cases the body's management intelligence is capable of turning on itself and thus destroying itself in a paradoxical and hopeless last ditch attempt to survive. This is rather like an animal caught in a trap biting its trapped leg off to gain its freedom only to later die of septicaemia or unable to defend itself from other prey animals.

This issue of the treatment itself being destructive is patently clear in the case of chemotherapy. This is hardly surprising as chemotherapy evolved out of mustard gas $C_4H_8Cl_2S$ Sulphur mustard. The connection is that mustard gas as used in WWI was found to destroy white blood cells. Consequently it was engineered to destroy cancer cells, now widely known to destroy not just cancerous cells but healthy cells thus also damaging the immune system.

Since the start of the pharmaceutical profession proper it has emerged that all medications are poisonous and all poisons are potential medicines. Many medical solutions are therefore essentially treating one trauma by traumatising the body and its cells with a secondary chemical trauma, plus a list of further and subsequent chemical traumas all piggy-backing on the previous one. All this is under the premise of well meaning intentions to heal the original problem. Whatever happened to Hippocrates' advice of "do no harm?"

There are a growing number of doctors who are not happy with this situation. Now there is a growing trend to find alternative solutions for their patient's treatment. A popular development is the use of new extracts being found in common and exotic or tropical plants. Those treatments claimed to be ideal for fighting cancer, are reported to have at least as good if not better life expectancy than chemotherapy. One important aspect is they conform to Hippocrates' advice and "do no harm." Thus there are apparently few if any uncomfortable and traumatic side effects. The spinoff bonus is the patient's immune and innate healing systems remain intact and capable to fight on.

This leaves us with an interesting question about the efficacy of these homeopathic treatments. As they are unlikely to be healing the underlying emotional trauma, are they then reactivating the switched off senescence programs, which then allow the cells beliefs, values, identity and purpose programming to function properly again?

The biggest bonus of all these natural alternatives is possibly the reason why they are proving to be effective. The first possibility is the fact they are natural substances and thus the body's innate healing intelligence may recognise and therefore work with them far better than the synthesized chemical poisons passed off by the pharmaceutical companies as beneficial medicines. However natural plant remedies work, this does not address the problem of any background emotional causal problems being dealt with. This may be reflected in the fact the plant extracts contain natural substance based messaging factors capable of inducing the body's natural innate emotional stress relieving hormones and neurotransmitters to be effective. Is this all part of the same intelligence as Dr Deepak Chopra refers to as the body's own pharmacy having the instructions within the treatment itself? Furthermore, the intuitive sensitivity of the doctors prescribing these natural substances may be the basis of a support telepathic message with the patient's innate healing systems. This likely indicates the doctor is mindful to care with minimal interference with the principal message of "doing no harm." Thus inadvertently the doctor is supporting the patient in resolving their deep emotional trauma without either of them realising.

Hippocrates stated that "a patient might recover from belief in the goodness of the physician." This seems to have turned a full 180° and now patients may not recover for the fear of the horrors the physician might inflict upon them with prescription poisons. Please note Hippocrates clearly says 'belief,' meaning an acceptance that something exists or is true, in this case based on experience and possibly intuitive confidence. Faith is based on spiritual or emotional conviction rather than scientific proof. This is likely the irrational basis for the term faith healing, which could more appropriately be called placebo healing. Though the meaning of belief and faith may ultimately only have subtle differences, despite misuse, the subconscious centres of intelligence are highly sensitive to those differences. However large or small, they are all important. There is one more element to this argument; confidence based on trust is the psychological experience element, which provides the necessary proof that in turn enables the psychological placebo effect to work. The danger is that if that trust is sufficiently dented or broken the entire belief or faith placebo effect may collapse like a house of cards.

It goes without saying that these new age doctors must do their diagnosis and prescribe treatment as appropriate. What also may be happening is the fact, if the telepathic message indicates the treatment is neither toxic nor in any other way dangerous, the innate healing system is then primed and already willing and able to work with the treatment rather than blocking it. If this does not happen then the underlying emotional issues remain to be healed. If this does not happen especially where they are the cause of the emotional imbalance sufficient to trigger cells to become cancerous, the inevitable end is that cancer will eventually win for no more valid reason than default. This may account for the reason cancers regarded to be in remission following chemotherapy and other treatments, stubbornly reappear.

Obviously treating the emotional traumas within the intelligence systems of cells, glands, organs, and other bodily parts also within the emotional intelligence itself, is going to require a very special form of alternative support healing. As such, if this is true, I understand why within my alternative support healing, as with orthodox medicine's well practiced procedures, just one error or omission let alone a multitude of them can spoil or block innate healing. This appears to be, at least one answer to the question why treatment works for some and not for others. This also explains that all forms and degrees of errors represent unnecessary interference. For these reasons, I believe it is so important to understand at the very least the principles of the body and its intelligence systems. Ultimately they are incredibly capable but also immensely vulnerable to well meaning but the wrong help.

All this further demonstrates that like the man whose eye mal-performed due to one tiny muscle, just one small error can change so much and thus disrupt us from working effectively. Herein lies the complexity, finesse and sensitivity required of support healing. That shouts out loudly this specific form of support healing at least works following orthodox treatment. This leaves us with the notion that at its very best, it may be regarded as a parallel team process within the overall orthodox medical box of solutions.

I am sure we all experience how the wrong choice of just one word in an explanation can change the dynamics of a love relationship, a family argument or perhaps a career move interview. Another area I have noticed this effect is when asking a question at a conference. While intending to focus on one issue, just one wrong or inappropriate word ends up side-tracking the answer into quite a different area. If this happens, one is not always able to ask the question a second time. This indicates how and why life coaching gives such importance to word associations. Not only do they have powerful links to emotional stress and stressor aftermaths but also each listener is making their unique new emotional connections by virtue of their own special understanding of the meaning and nuances of those words. This is seen in the process of writing or altering computer programs. Just one error in thousands of letters and symbols can change the desired result or simply block it from working at all.

Whether it is radiation, hazardous chemicals or a serious emotional issue, they are all traumas to the mind and body for, which only the emotional intelligence understands. This is the fundamental reason why within the healers mind, there must never be the slightest idea, suggestion, intent or action beyond being at service to the direction of the patient's innate healing intelligent and its guidance.

Only the innate healing system intelligence can know and understand all the complexities of all the mind's processes involved in any particular health condition. For this reason it is only the innate healing intelligence that knows and fully understands exactly what the ideal healing should and will be.

Due to their training, alternative healers have a predominance to lay their hands on the patient as beholden to faith and spiritual healing tradition. They are taught to move their hands over the patient's body as an act of clearing away disturbed energy and thus leading to healing. Quite what difference this method would have made to any of the cases mentioned in the general text or in the case histories section is clearly beyond my understanding. I already mentioned that freeing up blocked energy meridians is exactly what acupuncturists do. Acupuncture is an extremely detailed documented therapy. Get the needles in the wrong place and there is no benefit. By virtue of their demanding training, acupuncturists understand precisely what they are doing and always careful to do no harm.

I have made a point of watching spiritual healers at healing displays and have tested such training myself. I am certain few have little idea what they are doing or how their actions could possible induce healing. The process can be appropriate in some cases. I agree it does induce a sense of mild relaxation to the patient. However, where I have seen it used as a deliberate form of healing, it breaks my rule of non-interference. I recognise the fact that some medical institutions believe the practice to be conducive to the overall healing process. This at least shows a willingness to match alternative support healing with orthodox medicine. This is the point I make about teamwork. However, the fact is that close attention of this type in a calm atmosphere by any trusted person whether a healer or not will naturally induce an equivalent sense of ease. This in no way suggests it is without any value at all. Being at ease, our body is more capable of healing itself. This is largely because we are not feeding it with stress cortisol, which weakens the immune and innate healing systems and much more.

High performing life coaching is more effective when the coach intuitively asks questions though not understanding the significance of the questions or even individual words their client uses. It is within this process that only the perfect information is telepathically transferred to the patient's innate healing intelligence. The reason why this is necessary is the same as explained earlier, in that emotional traumas of trying to help may block the innate healer from functioning until the patient has consciously recognised and dealt with the underlying trauma or traumas. This deepens the explanation of why life coaching can be useful for the alternative support healer.

In my work of discovering how my support healing worked; especially concerning healing cancers; it came to my attention that cells have aging systems known medically as senescence or aging programs. Cancers are known to develop in cells that have had their self regulating senescence programs turned off. Normally, the process of healthy cell aging slows their rate of dividing until eventually they achieve apoptosis or programmed death. When senescence programs are somehow turned off, the cells may form into benign tumours. Without this vital aging senescence information in an active state, Dr. Deepak Chopra says, *"cells become unregulated, formless and chaotic."*

These now rogue cells without their senescence aging program enter what is known as a state of immortality. This means they do not age and die naturally. Instead they perpetuate and divide rapidly quickly developing a tumour.

University research programs and pharmaceutical companies are searching for ways to chemically switch those dormant senescence programs back on again. While this is undoubtedly the sensible path to take, one wonders what diabolical pharmaceutical concoctions will be devised in the process that will cause additional traumas to the body.

I do not and would not advocate direct support healing before medical involvement. At least this has the advantage of the patient having a basic understanding of what their problem really is. This is therefore also, a starting point for the support healer to work from.

One such case was of a boy who had been undergoing regular dialysis treatment at Great Ormond Street children's Hospital in London. For unknown reasons to the hospital staff, the latest dialysis was having no effect; consequently he was slipping into a coma. I was called in urgently and minutes after I left the hospital the boy made a remarkable recovery as the dialysis began working as expected. Therefore, it appears that orthodox medical support backed up with my method of support healing to the patient's emotional and innate healing intelligence systems can apparently be the difference that makes a difference but yes, there is no factual or medical proof.

Some patient's arrived with very negative beliefs of the "shooting own foot" type. This was often expressed in comments like, *"I know you have helped other people but I doubt you can heal me."* I am sure this negative self-talk would do little to help any telepathic connections preceding the healing. Negative beliefs or faith carry negatively charged energy, which in turn support negative or blocking information intelligence. As such negative faith is another form of stress further depressing the immune system, and it is clear it does little good. Once I realised the greater significance of the two sides of emotional energy, it was obvious negative faith has to be spotted and resolved before any other healing can begin. This is always important as negative faith is pure and simply another form of emotional interference albeit from within the patient. As the patient is ultimately their own best healer this is an important point to resolve.

There are various processes within NLP and life coaching ideally suited to dealing with this problem. In a nut shell this is supplying the right information to the right parts at the right and same time. Hypnosis or deep meditation may not work in these cases because the negative self-talk convinces the patient nothing will work.

Apart from people's habits of instantly jumping to wrong conclusions, the fastest thing I know of in the body/mind is telepathy, emotional intelligence hormones and neurotransmitters. When telepathy passes the right information to the right parts at the same time, all these are combined by the body/mind in the most appropriate order, and thus healing from the inside can be exceedingly fast.

As unnecessary hormones and neurotransmitters released by traumas are ultimately responsible for switching active senescence programs off, switching cancer cell senescence programs back on again can possibly only happen by another hormone shock. The question is then how to create the perfect anti-trauma shock, which results in the perfect reverse process managed by one or more centres of healing intelligence within the patient. Perhaps chemotherapy and other anti-cancer drugs that do so much damage in the process, that they become this anti-trauma trauma. Although this may be correct in all those cancer cases I was involved in, there was no anti-trauma shock. Therefore something else was at work in a far more subtle way.

Some doctors know this can happen for no accountable reason and is referred to as spontaneous healing. When this happens naturally it can only be via an emotional shift necessarily releasing whatever is needed to switch those vital senescence programs back on again.

Therefore, there must be an additional factor or a completely different set of factors to make up the perfect innate healing package.

Whatever the truth, that can only be via the release of the right hormones, neurotransmitters or other body chemicals with the perfect messaging or programming information essential to reverse the rogue programming and switch those programs back on again. By the example of the inadvertent release of bodily chemicals, we see how an emotional trauma or simply one deeply troubling idea may cause any number of disturbed health conditions to happen within the body. Stress, stressors, pain, traumas and the unnecessary production of cortisol is an example of how an entire series of processes can be triggered by vulnerability to one hurtful word or just seeing or even sensing an existing or a new emotional stressor. The resultant emotions with their modified stressed intelligence then activate a sequence of glands causing them to release hormones and neurotransmitters with peripheral consequences to our health and happiness beyond our awareness and thus beyond understanding. Somewhere in that process is the key to my support healing.

Despite medical science's enormous capabilities, researchers know in many cases they are still only scratching the surface of how the human body and the brain work. BBC television aired a program showing some extraordinary events such as a man suffering severe concussion. He found after his recovery he had an incredible capability to spontaneously play wonderful melodies on the piano. Another man suffered a stroke and went into a coma. When he emerged from the coma he saw the world in geometric shapes and had a genius mind for mathematics. In one personal encounter, a young man suffered a high dose of radiation sufficient to kill him. Not only did he survive, after the accident he found he had the capability to paint stunning pictures, all depicting extraterrestrial planet landscapes.

Medical researchers fully understand the innate healing system exists. The problem is it is almost unfathomable because it is pure intelligence and it is in every cell. This is to say; there is no independent structure to dissect by any means. Therefore, there is no method of tapping into it and recording it in its entirety for the purpose of replicating it. We can only observe it at work as in cases of observing spontaneous healing after the event.

While this scenario is understandable, newly driven to learn about causes and effects; I found myself apparently doing what I had learnt was taboo, intrusive and interfering. As the healings I was faced with were becoming more and more challenging it became evident; in creating the best rapport, it was important to understand the medical complications of an illness. That meant understanding the patient's medical treatment. This proved to be a development not a setback resulting in intrusive interference. I found this was because this level of understanding highlighted the body's resistance and that meant there had to be another issue, which could only be emotional blockages. The need to understand was clarified as understanding what the doctors were trying to achieve and how. This meant there was an advantage in me choosing, which combination of NLP, life-coaching and or support healing to use. On occasions all merged into one continuous intuitive and telepathic flow of the perfect energy, information and non-interference. When this happened I never failed to be amazed at the incredible intelligence and knowhow of this life force emanating from one apparently fragile spark of life.

I have no evidence or proof only a theory that once orthodox treatment has failed, a part of the medical treatment may remain in the patient's body. Thus, once the emotional blockage is cleared that prescribed medication is possibly still able to support the body's innate healing system intelligence in aiding the final healing.

To understand how NLP and life coaching work is to recognise these are the formalisation of natural processes of effective interrogation. It is then hardly surprising that I find the same quality within my own support healing. The word interrogation seems a harsh, almost brutal process for such a seemingly delicate subject as healing. Interrogation is how we acquire information from another person. If interrogated at the conscious level, the interrogator gets largely what the interrogated wants to be believed, which may be equally fact or fiction. NLP and life coaching naturally interrogates at the subconscious level. Because the subconscious cannot lie or create fictitious accounts it divulges the truth and only the truth.

I mentioned earlier that best intentions are invariably full of errors and that just one error is one error too many. It is therefore when considering this vital quality of support healing that I accept the word interrogation is what must be; so there are no errors or interference. Another coach or healer may prefer the word, questioning or conversation, another gentler soul may feel the words "pussy footing" more appropriate so not to frighten their client into mind freeze. To my mind that is neither NLP nor life coaching therapy, it is wilful interfering due to the presumption as to what is best. This just goes to show how we all apply different nuances to words, which no doubt reflect each individual's character and how well they know themselves thus the quality of the results they get.

Whatever the word the formalisation of coaching has been and continues to be a process by which the life coach understands precisely how to ask the perfect question and following questions that will act upon the patient's subconscious awareness. Out of the millions of brain connections the perfect solution then comes from the patient's subconscious intelligence and is intuitively transferred to their conscious awareness.

I said, "Life coaching is a formalisation of a natural process of mind processes." When I began studying NLP and life coaching, it was three decades after starting my support healing. From this experience I realised I had naturally been interrogating my patients in a coaching manner from the beginning of using my healing gift. This was about the same time as NLP was being formalised and almost certainly before life coaching was standardised or became a widely adopted profession as it is today.

Both in life coaching and NLP therapy it is recognised that a close rapport with the coachee or patient is important if not essential for success. This rapport proved to be the same intuitive and telepathic connection as I refer to in the case of support healing. Further analysis of this intuition revealed that intuition could only be via a telepathic connection between my patient and myself. Therefore, the process of creating a positive rapport is essential not just with the conscious but certainly with the subconscious mind.

A perfect example of this process is explained further on in the case of a mature woman who had suffered continuous stomach pain since her early teens. No doctor had been able to find the cause or even a psychosomatic remedy that worked. Yet, in a few minutes of my intuitive interrogation at the start of the healing session, her pains stopped and vanished.

My conclusion is that I became so familiar with following intuitive and telepathic conversations they happened naturally and easily as though it was quite unextraordinary so creating that perfect rapport that passed unnoticed. It transpires that this almost mundane easy telepathic conversation had its reason in the patient opening up to the necessary subconscious conversation. This was not that I, as the support healer could know everything about my patient. This was so the patient could willingly lower their inner shields, barriers and emotional defences so their centres of intelligence that had been divided by emotional trauma, could connect again.

In the above case, this telepathic conversation broke the ice and the previously immovable obstructions melted the instant she had made her subconscious emotional connections. In a few moments of this rarefied atmosphere, she understood and healed something inside she had actually long known about. Only for emotional reasons, she could not or would not accept whatever happened. This last point illustrates that we can be consciously aware of our emotional hang-ups causing pain but not be prepared to go that extra mile to resolve them. This case suggested to me that she suffered her own subconscious trauma that triggered the, "want to but cannot" syndrome.

I can only conclude the reason why over the years of this woman's perpetual pain, no treatment worked, whether provided by a doctor of psychotherapists was for one reason. This was the fact they were trying to intervene in something she was simply albeit subconsciously, not prepared to approach emotionally thus setting up a virtual barrier to treatment. Analysis of this case suggests somewhere along the line she had completed the emotional healing all by herself. That was when she stepped outside of her comfort zone to ask for help. Similar to Mark, the racing driver, I was called upon to facilitate the final part of that emotional healing. This appears to be providing the perfect key, in a precise form although I will never consciously be able to explain or understand the fine details of how it worked.

Neither my alternative support healing nor life coaching or NLP seeks to control, inform or give good counsel. The purpose is to move the coachee's or patient's awareness out and away from being stuck in the problem space and then into their unique solution or healing space. This is very much if not entirely a subconscious mind process. The life coach will never understand or know so much as a fraction of what their coaching has moved inside their client's mind and subconscious reasoning. The fact is that even the client or coachee themselves have little idea of what has changed. All they are aware of is the intuitive understanding of what they can do to change their situation from stuck to the performance they had previously been failing to achieve. I believe this is demonstrated by the case of the man emerging from a coma to find he had a previously unknown and amazing talent for playing the piano.

During my NLP basic and masters training I encountered several doctors on the courses. They were there because they had discovered that NLP and life coaching style interrogation was quicker and more reliable than traditional medical diagnosis. Consequently NLP and life coaching therapy could be as good as or even better than placebo sugar pills. Therefore, if the doctor is also a trained life coach and they support the release of any emotional blockages both conscious and subconscious within the patient; then as suggested above; whatever the innate healing intelligence that is blocked, it is then freed and the patient is capable of self-healing.

In parallel to understanding the primary healing aspect of my healing gift, this awareness of how the brain/mind/body works, became key to creating new high performance management programs. These were designed to replace old redundant programs that are creating their own problems rather than performing as they had done before. For example, I could see that new brain management programs were needed for controlling levels of stress that few of our ancestors knew anything about. Therefore, it is hardly surprising we have no evolved defences to protect us from stress overwhelm and burnout.

Charles Darwin introduced Evolution and the Origin of Species to the world back in 1859. Since then neuroscience and medical sciences have gradually improved our knowledge of how evolution controls and changes information and energy. Charles Darwin demonstrated that DNA evolution is constantly on the move in reprogramming itself according to changing circumstances or environments. What is clear is that process is far too slow to meet the speed and the need of modern performance demands. Therefore, we need a helping hand to literally leap-frog our DNA programming beliefs and subconscious performance parameters into the 21st Century. This is the field of developing subconscious automatic high performance such as we see in top sports people. The process could be described as sidelining outdated underperforming DNA behaviours and replacing them with new programs specifically designed to accommodate performance levels required by modern competitive standards for the precise purpose of winning.

During the past decade the study of cell senescence programming has grown a mainstream following in medical research. This area of interest is not yet proven definitively, though it does give a greater understanding of why cells become cancerous and they do not die in the normal manner. One aspect of the senescence programs demonstrates that as intelligent as the body/mind is, it has its own shortcomings. In brief, this is one reason why we have a need for doctors, hospitals, surgeons, therapists, life coaches and indeed alternative support healers.

Part of my involvement in this line of research was to learn about the various hormones and neurotransmitters produced by the body that act as messengers and switching devices. Medical research has shown how those processes effect behaviour from the changes in our thoughts right down to the behaviour of single muscles to groups of cells. The nub of this point is that hormones and neurotransmitters transfer intelligent information from environmental influences to thought and emotional energy and then into physical energy and performance. This transfer from information to the physical plane may occur in seconds or over decades.

Because innate healing intelligence is in every cell and every cell is in constant communication with all other cells there is a stream of information feeding centres of healing intelligence. Those centres of intelligence direct healing information via neurotransmitters to where it is needed. Therefore in order to further understand any successful healing therapy process; it was necessary to first get to know how inner intelligence and channels of information can be blocked. Once that was ascertained then it became clearer how the innate healing solution may be activated. In understanding and rationalising all the above, it became apparent how impossible this task is. Yet when any healing worked it is evidently exactly that process that had been activated. Hence, we get back to the fact that understanding what the process is, is one thing but then there is absolutely no need for the support healer to interfere because the patient's innate healing intelligence already knows all that is needed to be understood. So why should the support healer need to understand? My conclusion is that in understanding but not interfering, a critical subconscious confidence is possible, which opens the door to a dynamic telepathic communication between the patient and support healer leading to the healing process.

Though we do not realise the fact, telepathic communication is permanently switched on. The question is where is that communication being received? What must be understood is that any ideas the healer has and believes to be helpful are instantly transmitted to the patient's innate healing intelligence. I believe that any such information the innate healing intelligence finds to be unhelpful is classified as interference and so the communication link between the support healer and the patient is shut down or not opened. Furthermore the patient intuitively recognises that nothing has been healed and may also experience an emotional sense of frustration.

Growing conclusions indicate that emotional intelligence is not only important it is also more powerful than previously understood. In this book I address how emotional intelligence can be tricked into triggering unnecessary hormones like cortisol. Consequently, if emotional intelligence is not being addressed correctly, it appears to be capable of morphing into a resisting force as in blocking its own healing information or releasing a self destructive force. One such process is the switching off of cell senescence programs that subsequently result in tumours.

In the event that a support healer forcibly projects limiting ideas perceived to be helpful, the resultant blocking effect could feasibly aggravate an already delicate situation. This may occur where the support healer becomes emotionally involved with the patient in the sense of wanting them to be healed. That may happen for instance, where a support healer feels the terrible injustice of the patient's condition. That is already a slippery slope to interfering.

If interfering begins the process of releasing limiting hormones and neurotransmitter messaging, the result is to block treatment rather than manifesting as a healing energy and intelligence. Therein may lay another explanation why specific medications, orthodox medical treatment also many attempts by alternative healing or other therapists, do not always work as expected or hoped for. A case in mind was the woman with stomach pains that no doctor or psychotherapist could resolve. Consequently, there is a case for suggesting all types of healing therapies would improve their effectiveness by learning how to address any obvious or hidden emotional issues. This may be manifest in being sensitive and sympathetic to their client's emotional balance but not interfering, before beginning their treatment. Being sensitive and sympathetic without interfering is to say, expressing the observation of a disturbed energy and then let the client freely release their emotional feelings if they are ready to do that. The refinement of this natural healing process is in being sympathetic without offering good advice. It is guaranteed that any advice even if solicited by the client, is interfering in something the therapist cannot understand.

To demonstrate this, the basis of this book is very much underlined on tried and tested conclusions. Like most other people I have been challenged with three particularly important developments. One is chronic hay fever, which blighted every summer from the age of six. Another has been stress burnout and the other arthritic gout arrived after burnout in my mid fifties and is likely to have been triggered by the burnout trauma. All these plagued my life until I began to understand how I was responsible for them. Ninety nine percent of the hay fever turned out to be due to my diet and not the spring, summer and autumn pollen or fungal spores. It was not until my mid forties that I discovered the truth. After a life time of sneezing my way through school, sports, college and exams or being numbed by antihistamines of every description, size and colour, it all turned out to be my own fault. The moment I removed all wheat, yeast and many but not all milk products from my diet; despite the pollen still being present; the hay fever and the sneezing stopped.

The fact was, I was not allergic to pollen neither was I allergic to wheat or milk products. The truth is my body has an inherent intolerance to these recognised staple foods. This intolerance produces elevated levels of body inflammation, which causes the body to produce histamine, which in turn raises my sensitivity to pollens, dusts and fungal spores. This process appears to be augmented by higher summer temperatures also by humidity. These two things are relatively easy to understand. What is less apparent is why certain locations which have the same pollens can have different influences. Aggravating this intolerance on a daily basis by breakfasting on toast or cereals caused my body to sustain permanent high body inflammation. This raised my sensitivity and wore down my immune system. The result was in also being susceptible to every winter, spring, summer or autumn cold and flu germ that I bumped into. When I found my eating behaviours and habits that weakened my system and stopped doing those things, this aspect of high susceptibility changed dramatically.

The reason I mention this is to demonstrate how in life we all can do so much we believe to be good but in fact we are doing the worst thing possible. In managing my business diligently, working long hours and giving my all, I believed this was a good performance strategy and the resultant successes seemed to be the proof of the pudding. Well yes, until; like the hay fever caused by eating the wrong foods, burnout adequately showed me how all the time I had been storing up stress to the point my body/brain intelligence systems could no longer tolerate my behaviours.

So far, I got off lightly. That burnout crisis could have so easily been sudden death syndrome or morphing into cancer. This does not mean I am traumatised by what did not happen and it does not mean I rap myself up in cotton wool. I still push myself when necessary and do not balk at unexpected effort. What I do, do is to take a little more notice of myself so that I get the job done without any untoward stress or other downside consequences.

Finding the solution to my health intolerances changed how I look at challenges of all types and degree. Now, most of all; I am quick to take careful notice of intuition, my feelings intelligence and anything that could be the slightest guidance from my subconscious intelligence. It could be regarded as the wisdom that comes with age and experience. This is I believe, too simplistic as we all can go through life blinded by what we do not understand. A friend who suffers with pollen and animal fur, point blank refuses to even test my discoveries for himself. A few days ago I heard of another person who did exactly as I did and they too stopped their crippling summer hay fever without the need for antihistamines. I have shared this discovery with many people so afflicted and have been amazed to find their breakfast cereals, toast, sandwiches and more are more important than respecting their own bodies, general health and comfort. What surprises me most is that doctors know about this intolerance factor but for some bizarre reason seem to keep it to themselves. They prefer to prescribe antihistamines rather than properly sharing details with their patients as to the real and simple cause and solution. It is not just that grain products in combination with baker's yeast cause heightened inflammation and histamine, these and other foods are toxic to my body therefore depleting and exhausting its defences and energy.

When I developed arthritic gout, I began to search for what I was doing to cause each crisis. Research revealed that the old fairy story of inherited kidney weakness was not the problem. This is a widely believed piece of misinformation, which results in the use of some fairly dangerous pharmaceutical treatments. As with hay fever it proved to be some foods that are the catalysts but not all the time. Seasonal changes, humidity and temperature changes are now recognised as prime activators. Certainly a gout crisis can be quickly aggravated by specific foods and beverages, notably those high in purines. The liver turns the purines into uric acid in such quantities that perfectly healthy kidneys (traditionally blamed for the gouty arthritis) cannot cope, therefore excess uric acid remains in the blood stream. As levels of uric acid rise the needle like crystals in the acid get stuck in big toe joints causing painful swelling. Although referred to as simply arthritis, the same uric acid crystals may cause swelling of finger, hand, knee, ankle and other joints. In the early days because I did not know better, I resorted to prescribed pills. When I discovered the consequences after long term use of that medication and its side effects, I began looking for a better solution by understanding the problem as fully as possible. From then on I devoted my efforts to prevention rather than curing. When in severe discomfort it is natural that we want to relieve the pain as soon as possible. Consequently I focus more on knowing myself and keeping my body healthy rather than undermining it through ignorance.

Like many people under permanent stress, as my work load and worries grew, I began suffering with persistent headaches and increasing migraine attacks. This meant I virtually lived on a diet of paracetamol or other pain killers or simply suffered. Once I got the hay fever controlled, surprisingly; for the first time I looked into the reason for headaches and migraine. Yes, there it was the same culprit and foe high body inflammation.

Because headaches and migraine were a common thing, I had never made the connection with eating dark chocolate. Once I understood the intolerance factors, I was also able to confirm dark chocolate as a culprit able to rapidly increase inflammation in a specific way that resulted in either a headache or migraine.

I found my body intolerance to various foods was aligned with increasing age. My research indicated that my body was always intolerant of those foods but in my younger days my body had a better and more rapid capability in overcoming those intolerance effects. Because these intolerances are in fact forms of stress, this gives us more understanding of why stress levels and body inflammation are closely connected. Naturally one train of thought leads to others. Discussing my discoveries with a homeopathic pharmacist I learnt of one natural plant extract that I now take regularly, which lowers body inflammation, which decreases any risks of producing histamine and has put an end to all headaches and migraines. A few drops daily of an extract from the common blackberry bush buds known as Ribies Nigrum Mac BG, proved to be a highly effective preventative treatment. With zero danger or side effects and costing a few pennies daily, not mega bucks as the case of complex medications.

The question then arose as to why my innate healing intelligence had not done its job. With the advent of more study and analysis, I realised that my innate healing intelligence had been doing its job. When it became overloaded it screamed for help in the form of headaches, migraine, high histamine production and hay fever attacks also later on gouty arthritis. In its own way it had been doing its best to bring to my attention to the fact that, it was my habitually presumed healthy eating habits that were causing these intolerance problems.

The resultant dilemma was how I could understand what my innate healing intelligence wanted to convey without having to suffer first? To find the answers entailed monitoring exactly what effect any one or combinations of intolerant foods had. Without the guidance of a medical professional who understands these issues, there is no way to learn these simple remedies especially when the medical profession prefer to prescribe the easy option of antihistamines.

Until we learn by experience or good fortune, it seems to be our lot to suffer until we wake up, start learning how to listen to our inner intelligence and getting better at knowing ourselves particularly how our body intelligence communicates with our conscious awareness.

Today there are no excuses as so much information is freely available on the internet on practically any subject imaginable. Though undertaking some personal research in this way, there is the distinct probability that the information turns into overload especially as so much information can appear contradictory. My solution to this problem was to take one issue at a time and research it as fully as I was able to do via verifiable sources.

I have referred to many talented also extremely knowledgeable people and their own books dealing with the inner healer or associated subjects. Also I recount meaningful real life stories that help to explain more of the process of mind and body. Observing ourselves is certainly important to our successes. Stories passed down through generations were how sound guidance was passed on to new generations. In modern high speed, high stress cultures with divorce broken families and thus missing parental guidance, much of that style of trickle down information has largely disappeared.

To some extent useful anecdotes and the unwritten advice has now been documented on websites but relatively few of us get to read those. However a modern method of sharing information has evolved as the old slid into disuse. Films and now notably animated films directed at children invariably convey sound advice previously shared by bedtime stories. Those messages are quite clear for children and there are also stories for adults, although they tend to be carefully camouflaged. Spotting the messages is somewhat similar to noticing subconscious intuition or telepathic messaging.

I recall the film "Good Will Hunting, starring Robin Williams and Matt Damon. Matt Damon plays the role of a brilliant young man, Will Hunting who has serious emotional and behavioural problems blocking his relationships with people, as well as his enormous potential career prospects. What makes the film and story more fascinating is its subliminal theme. This is the story of how and why our success beliefs, values and behaviours become distorted by emotional traumas.

Robin Williams plays the psychologist, who finally pulls Will Hunting's emotional trigger. Matt Damon's character Will Hunting considered himself safe behind his purpose built alternative-reality shielding. In the film he is taken by surprise as Robin Williams throws a left hook to Matt Damon's vulnerable soft emotional underbelly. Shaken, he is faced with his real reality. With nowhere to hide, he finally accepts himself as he really is. Robin Williams ruthlessly pursues his advantage by pushing Will Hunting to face what has to change in order to gain the thing he most wants but had been frightened of the consequences and had been running from for most of his life. Will Hunting let's go of his protective shield as he begins to heal a deep emotional scar.

The twist in this tale is that Will Hunting's reaction at being uncovered is to turn agent provocateur. Demonstrating his level of intelligence and fast learning skills, he had observed exactly what the psychotherapist had done and how. He takes his revenge by immediately and brutally lifting the lid off the psychologist's own internal emotional blockage.

This is an important life story that not only affects us all but shows how and why everyone with the correct training can be a support healer especially when we understand the boundaries of intervening and not interfering. If we are prepared to accept it, it gives us, the opportunity to take a look at ourselves. This is; if we can be open to recognising our own protective shields and then even take a peek at the unnecessary emotional baggage of reality distortions we have inadvertently collected and purposefully or accidentally used to create our own purpose built stumbling blocks. Daring to do this, we may find all the false beliefs, and smoke screen values preventing us to achieve what really matters - that is who we really are and what we are really capable of accomplishing if only we will allow ourselves to do all that comes to light.

Having the fortitude to open our emotional cupboards and look inside, we may in those moments heal some things that had been causing problems elsewhere for a very long time. The most effective way to do this is to find a good life coach. The reason this is important is that those emotional blockages prevent us from self recognising whatever we are hiding from. The only problem is, in the case of some complex emotional issues, they require a specific process, which respects how the mind and emotional intelligence works. Then stuck issues can be brought to the surface by a life coach into the light without causing more harm or slamming the door shut again.

In one scene Will Hunting is in a bar listening to a university student trying to impress a pretty girl with what he passes off as his own intellect and knowledge. Will Hunting unmasks the young man's plagiarised knowledge, by quoting all the books from which that information had been lifted, Damon then says to the young man: *"Don't you have any original thoughts of your own?"*

I found this fascinating and consider we should all ask ourselves this question and never stop doing so. What are our original thoughts and where are they? How do we come by them or where, even why are they ignored, buried or are we hiding from them? If those we choose to adopt are not ours, whose are they and why are they so important. Why do we allow our original creative thoughts and ideas capable of releasing our own genius to be sidelined by the beliefs of others? Are we frightened of our own thoughts, if so why? Alternatively, why do we follow our own limiting ideas especially if they do not work for us?

Answer these questions and we begin to see precisely who we aspire to be, who we currently are and why we have so many lost or abandoned dreams destined to wither on the vine or cause our lives to be more complex or difficult than need be. All this is only because we do not have a works manual as to how to manage our own brain also the amazing agglomeration of systems that keep our whole life force and its balanced functioning in the best working order.

The fortunate ones may grow up guided by elders whether family or perhaps school and university who understand these important principles and take the time to share those. If not, we have little option than to learn about the wheel of life and success by unnecessarily reinventing it by trial, error and constantly falling over ourselves and wondering why we rarely seem to get it right.

In this modern world we are likely to get a barrage of lies, deliberate marketing misinformation, half truths and fake news. Other than our own limited influence groups, there are few guide lines as to how to make a difference, thus we get ourselves caught in a set of limiting behaviour and thinking patterns. How much we know about ourselves is one good example of this limiting process. Self motivation for success demands that we make the effort to understand the enormous wealth of intelligence controlling how our brain and body works. Only by searching for and sharing this knowledge will the veils of ignorance and self-limitation be pushed aside so all can see the intelligence available within ourselves and how to access and use it to ensure we all succeed.

To answer all the above questions the addition of close examination of ancestors, their locations and professions, achievements, their beliefs and values may be helpful. Therefore, we begin to understand the impact and importance of subliminal influence on personal identity, image, function, capabilities, objectives, goals and dreams for the future and finally performance and much more. This is all about how good we are at knowing ourselves sufficiently to recognise our unique thoughts. Thus allowing ourselves to better create future objectives and goals synonymous with who we are now and the person we want to be in the future. While doing this, if we are open to intuitive and telepathic support, we may not waste so much of our time and energy with frivolous pipe dreams and unnecessary mistakes. This is in particular reference to unnecessarily reinventing the wheel of life especially if it happens to be the wrong wheel for our best potential performance.

The more we know, recognise and take meaningful notice of ourselves, and thus quickly deal with our emotional problems, the more we support our internal balance. It is not rocket science, all it takes is taking the time and effort to notice how so much internal intelligence is doing its best to point us in the right direction. All we have to do is seek the best guidance possible, open our eyes and minds to what has been staring us in the face but for redundant and limiting beliefs, we could not or would not recognise it.

Emotionally challenging issues we believe have been forgotten about for a long time, never die, they are just buried alive. Like the story of Will Hunting; resurrecting and freeing those issues has been sufficient for so many people to restart their healing systems when the most sophisticated medical treatment had failed. This speaks volumes about the damage and consequences we are capable of creating for ourselves. This is all for the sake of not knowing, not understanding who or what we really are or how we work.

Greater rewards are found when we deliberately search out and recognise which issues are still supporting us and which are either outdated or just plain redundant. How many of our behaviours and beliefs are frankly limiting our potential to succeed whether for health, family or profession? Which ones are creating unnecessary stress with all its secondary consequences? How many stumbling blocks do we create simply because we are too stubborn to be seen to be wrong?

The above is all relevant to the healing process because managing ourselves is no different than managing a business or indeed a country. Our beliefs and values have a profound effect on our health and in many cases blocking our innate healing intelligence. As living beings we may not become financially bankrupt but we are quite capable of bankrupting our own immune and innate healing systems due to stubborn ignorance or sheer arrogance.

As far as support healing is concerned, testing my findings and conclusions time and again has been principle in the investigation of continued further development of understanding the art of activating spontaneous healing. In the west most medical problems are treated after the build-up of discomfort, pain and crisis. Traditional Chinese and Indian medicines have a greater culture of focusing on balance and prevention. Acupuncture and martial arts from China reinforce the energy centres and their radiating meridians in the body in order to maintain a state of homeostasis. Yoga and ayurvedic medicine from India have the same principles at their roots. These ancient forms of medicine have also long had an eye on the importance of emotional balance as essential to health balance.

Famously, Dr Masura Emoto of Japan has demonstrated what negative emotional thoughts can do to ice crystals. In his books "The hidden Messages in Water" (1999), "The True Power of Water", and "The Secret Life of Water." he makes powerful arguments for maintaining emotional balance and particularly the energy of love for ourselves, for other people, our environment and nature in guarding our general health care. Considering the human body is comprised of roughly 85% water, his work illustrates how damaged, destabilised feelings, the wrong environments can seriously upset body balance and inner healing systems along with their intelligence centres.

Chapter 1

CASE HISTORIES

The following are case histories for the purpose of sharing a practical and experiential understanding of how the healing process works. In most cases names have been changed to respect confidentiality. In one case I use the real person's name such as the late Ninian Crichton-Stuart. Ninian was a patient more than 50 years ago. As a result of his healing experience he volunteered as a sponsor of many healing trips to Spain where he lived. He also recommended people to me in the UK as well as other countries much further afield. I have great pleasure to mention Ninian because I regard him as much a part of the support healing process as myself. In so many cases he was another key, which made the right connections. Ninian was responsible for persuading many people to ask for my assistance. It was through the intervention of Ninian and his trust in my support healing that many magical events of self discovery came to pass for so many people. Thus his accidental death while having an operation to remove a polyp, was a sudden, unexpected and tremendously sad loss.

It was Ninian who convinced the Spanish doctor who was given two weeks of freedom before being forced into hospital and intensive treatment to help him die with dignity. Why was this so special? It was because the doctor throughout his career in accordance with the law had been vehemently against spiritual and faith healers and actively denounced any he came across.

Ninian's case was one of cancer of the hip. When I first met him he was receiving medical treatment including chemotherapy. He came to see me because his doctor's latest prognosis was not good. Ninian was one of those who had no questions and no doubts. His was a trust in his intuitive awareness. Immediately after the healing session, Ninian said to me. *"You will not believe this but I actually felt something change in my leg during the healing. I have an intuitive impression this healing is going to work."*

Later he said that only after the healing did the cancer begin to go into remission and then disappear within a few weeks. My conclusion is that Ninian's and other people's similar experience, are in fact more than trust. When Ninian first spoke to me he was aware of a strong intuition the healing was going to work. Therefore, I ask the question, are we mistaking intuitive intelligence for more loosely used words such as faith or trust?

When reading the case histories and analyses please be careful to avoid making any immediate conclusions of your own. Each case is a snap shot on a much larger picture. It is only by means of steadily building a background of understanding and awareness that the larger picture of activating the body's healing begins to come into view.

Chapter 2

THE RACING CAR DRIVER

Ninian met me at Madrid airport; then drove us to an apartment somewhere in the centre of the city. Mark was my first patient of this healing trip, his pain was plainly etched deeply in his face, hands and fingers. I was introduced to a crumpled man reclining on an enormous armchair. The contorted position of his body spoke starkly of the agonizing pain he was enduring. I studied Mark lying there supported with an array of cushions tucked at all angles to give support to every part of his long suffering body.

Mark explained how he was driving a racing car until that devastating moment his world came to a shattering, traumatising halt and a state of limbo. His car crashed into a bridge at 200 mph. Now he was as crumpled, crunched and twisted as his car. Money was not a problem, despite asking surgeons around the world, none would touch him for fear of turning him into a permanent cripple or worse still, there was a risk of him dying on the operating table.

I stood in front of Mark in silence thinking what on earth am I doing here - what on earth can I do? I stared at him for what seemed an eternity but was really a minute or two, hoping for some inspiration. I didn't have a clue as to what I had to offer. What could I do for this poor soul? If ever there was a time for pulling something incredible out of the bag this was it. I had attended a course at a healing association school in England, to acquire an official healing certificate. The practical training was essentially related to moving stagnant energy with my hands. Clearly kneeling beside Mark moving his stagnant energy as also advised by the spiritual church healers who befriended me, was not going to fix this man's problems in a matter of seconds, minutes or even years of healing.

Just as I was letting go of any notion of what to do and admitting defeat, I realised I had quite naturally slipped into a mind state known by elite sports people as "the field" or "the Zone." The Zone is a state of letting go of conscious control and where the subconscious mind or inner intelligence takes full control. Spiritualists might call this being in a spiritual trance and hypnotherapists would describe this as a state of self hypnosis or hypnotic trance. Buddhists would call it a deep state of meditation or prana. The word prana means breath, though it also has connotations that come from Hinduism where the term prana or breath represents the concepts of life essence, soul and universal energy as a breath of embodiment.

I found myself looking deep into Mark's eyes focusing my thoughts to his subconscious mind.

My silent intuitive message to his subconscious and inner healing intelligence was this. *"What do you want me to do?"*

Everything was still. The room was silent like a stone. The next thing to happen was a calm, strong intuitive awareness. The deep visual and telepathic link broke and immediately I asked Mark to move to the nearby settee. I spoke the words aloud but with a strange unusual monotone voice. Mark looked at me in a way that could only be described as total disbelief; he didn't move a muscle. I repeated the same message. Then Mark said: *"Don't be a bloody fool, I can hardly move and anyway the pain would kill me."*

With no other response or any emotion, I repeated the same monotone message to move to the settee. Each time he complained, my voice become more demanding until Mark realised I was serious and was not about to change my mind. Eventually he rolled off his chair onto the floor. Agonisingly he crawled inch by inch on hands and knees to the settee. Finally, hunched up, the sweat of intense pain pouring down his face, almost crying he said, *"I cannot do any more."*

"Lay down on your stomach," I said.

The aggression and resistance now completely gone from his voice, Mark cried – *"I cannot, I'm in agony."*

Then I said: *"Mark I'm going to put you in a very deep state of relaxation where you may fall asleep. You don't have to say anything just do your best to work with me, think about letting go of the pain."*

Considering his physical pain, contrary to my expectations, the hypnotic induced relaxation took effect quickly. He entered a state of deep sleep as his body settled until lying flat.

I let him lay peacefully for a while. Then I noticed the unusual position of his spine. I was alarmed to see his lower backbone seemingly near breaking point was twisted in a sideways 'S' shape. Purely out of curiosity I placed my hands on his backbone, with my fingers barely touching him, at that instant his spine began to move. Within just a few seconds it was as straight as ever it had been. There was nothing else to do, my job was done. I waited a few minutes to see if any other changes occurred and then brought Mark back to a wakeful state. I advised him to lay still, and rest for a few minutes. Then I instructed him that when he felt ready and confident and sure there was no longer any pain he could sit up.

Mark opened his eyes, he lay still without saying a word then slowly he stirred himself. Dropping his legs over the edge of the settee he rolled into the sitting position. He hesitated for a few moments as he mentally checked himself for any pain. Then he gradually stood up. I remember sitting in that silence with Mark walking up and down the room for several minutes. To this day I have no idea what was going through his mind. Nothing was said and later Mark sat at the dining table with his wife, Ninian and myself as though it was dinner on a normal day in his life.

Mark was probably in some sort of state of shock. He said little throughout the dinner. More than likely trying to rationalise his feelings and emotions, not quite believing what had just happened. Ninian was in a calm confident and pleased mood, satisfied yet not at all surprised. Mark's wife made small talk and mostly just kept looking at Mark as though pinching herself so to wake up from a dream. For myself, there was a strange feeling, neither surprise, nor exhilaration, just a state of internal quietness. I knew I would think about this experience later. What had happened was certainly a shock for both Mark and his wife; they clearly needed to be alone to come to terms with what must have seemed unbelievable.

After the meal Ninian and I left heading south out of Madrid to our hotel. Then it was another day and the next patient. A week later I was back in the UK, Ninian called me after several days to say Mark was fine. A few weeks later he called again to say Mark was now playing golf twice a week. Ninian asked if it was alright for him to do that. I said he can do anything he likes so long as he stays away from racing cars.

I was puzzled by this case, even for me it was so quick and so remarkable that I began to think again about how the healing process worked. I had become used to many similar so called miracles of healing. Mostly these took time to confirm such as the disappearance of cancer needs tests and reports to finally confirm all was well. In Mark's case the evidence was clear and immediate.

From the beginning of my healing career I quickly had serious reservation about the idea of spiritual intervention or faith as a healing force. I really had no idea of my own as to who or what was the real healer. Mark was a landmark case where I had no doubt that he had healed himself. My part was all that was needed to unlock, release and push him to break through his limiting idea that he could not stand or walk without excruciating pain. At that moment I knew conclusively that could only happen once I had unconsciously taken instructions from Mark's inner or subconscious intelligence.

Sometime later I shared this story with an osteopath. He was not surprised as he explained how muscles have the ability to constrict themselves under shock or trauma and thus lock themselves in a painful position. He used the metaphor of the tab stops of an old fashioned type-writer still in general use at that time. Likewise, when traumatised muscles may lock in tension and are unable to release until the trauma program has been unlocked. The difficult part he said was to get the muscles to unlock their trauma program thus unlock themselves so they can freely move again.

Although the osteopath was sceptical that such a healing event could happen, his conclusion was that whatever did happen that day in Madrid, something caused Mark's muscle trauma to release itself. The osteopath's words were like a key turning in my mind. Was it the telepathic connection? Was it the physical process of moving from his safe chair onto the settee including the self drive to do that while suffering great pain? Was it the hypnosis and the combined relaxation? In a flash the bits of information about Mark tumbled into place. I was now absolutely certain that Mark really had healed himself. What's more, I was beginning to understand how. Added to that I began to realise what my part in the healing process had been. At that moment I had broad brush strokes of an awareness made up of flashes of understanding that my support healing was explainable by medical and neuroscience and had little if anything to do with fictitious beliefs of healing through spiritual entities. It was to take many more years and more apparent miracles of healing also the occasional failures to fully analyse and form a better understanding of how a complete healing process works.

Unravelling Mark's healing entailed understanding how the body and body/mind intelligence systems work. It is important to remember that the mind, body/mind's principle job is to protect itself by maintaining its natural state of homeostasis. It became apparent to me that if mind, brain, body/mind and its centres of intelligence do not like what we are doing or possibly what we are thinking of doing, planning or about to do, it uses emotions like doubt or fear to stop us from continuing. If that will not stop us then stronger action may be necessary to knock sense into us.

Also I have heard of some bizarre stories of unaccountable ways of some intelligent force stopping people from doing something that would lead them to harm. One such account was of a friend not being able to find his car key. The prolonged search eventually revealed the key in a pocket of a jacket he had worn the previous evening and had searched several times already. This delay made him late for his intended aeroplane. The plane crashed on landing in fog, killing all onboard.

Because I have heard of many similar events, I am not inclined to accept it was a pure coincidence. This man assured me he had searched the jacket pocket several times. Why his self survival intelligence had worked for him and the same had not happened for the other passengers or crew on that doomed flight, I cannot even begin to understand.

There was nothing Mark adored more than driving racing cars but with the passing years his reactions were just not quick enough. His personal fortune funded his driving to the extent his increasing age was overlooked. Through this experience it becomes clear the more we ignore our mental capacity to perform, ignore emotional and physical health and ignore those nagging intuitive reminders we are certain to head into disaster.

Mark knew he should stop but he loved the life and the adrenalin rush so he became stubborn always promising himself and his wife that he would retire next year. Well, we all know that like tomorrow, next year never comes. Something deeper in his emotional intelligence drove Mark on. It was the fear that retiring from driving was an unavoidable sign he was getting past his best, and that meant accepting that attached scary tag that he was getting old. After his accident Mark had plenty of time to reflect. The endless pain was a stark reminder of something he knew he should have stopped doing some time ago.

There is no proof but my experience of so many healings suggests that because Mark could not bring himself to stop driving. His survival and self protection intelligence did the only thing it could to stop him before he killed himself. The interesting fact is that despite the amazing distortion of his spinal cord, he came to no real or permanent harm. Once he accepted that decision he was ready to release himself. When I arrived on the scene, I simply started an internal process that led to Mark finishing the job of healing himself.

A similar thing occurred with a businessman who destroyed his own £12 million company. He blamed everyone in sight until finally realising that it was his own policies, strategies and stubborn determination against all advice that had destroyed his company. Only when he could recognise, accept and learn from his traumatic experience, was he able to start all over again.

After my intervention, Mark was up and running again, a little battered but, perhaps a great deal wiser also a lot safer now he was only driving small white golf balls down pristine fairways on a sun drenched Spanish golf course.

Chapter 3

CHRISTMAS AT HOME

This is a case that at first didn't seem to meet anyone's expectations. Jose's family were full of doubt and worry, especially as it was close to Christmas. Jose had serious cancer of the stomach. I arrived at Malaga airport where I was collected and taken to the Hospital where Jose was being cared for after his operation. The medical prognosis of a mass of secondary tumours was not encouraging, so false smiles and bravado was the order of the day. Though Jose was in reasonably good spirits, my feelings about his recovery were not good. Nevertheless my intuition told me there was something important for me to do so my effort and journey was not wasted.

Over time I have learnt to understand this type of intuition better. It is never clear what will happen. Intuitive guidance is to indicate that the effort is worthwhile; the long term result is not for me to know or judge. Everything is never as it appears on the surface; there is always more, a deeper story, a greater meaning and another step of evolution for us all.

Unlike English hospitals, healing was not permitted in Spain at that time. If caught I could have been in serious trouble. A mixture of care subterfuge and blatant lies by the family of my patients, avoided any questioning by the hospital staff. As I did not speak even basic Spanish, I could not be alone with Jose. This meant that I had to do my work while family and friends were coming and going, crying, greeting and chatting in his private room. The nursing staff were also popping in from time to time, busy doing their job. Slowly the staff became suspicious of this 'odd man out' that always seemed to be close to Jose but didn't speak any Spanish.

Intuitively I felt I should see Jose three times. This happened on successive days. On the third visit I was sure Jose would not last long. Now the chief nurse had asked who I was and what was I doing there. Fortunately I had already said my goodbyes. It was less than three weeks before Christmas. On my final visit, through my interpreter, I asked Jose - what do you want most of all? Without hesitation he said: *"To be at home with my family for Christmas."* Without thinking I replied "I'll see what I can do." "Consider it done," or some glib remark, all in the false bravado style of the day except intuitively I knew I meant it more seriously than I could ever explain in words. Finally almost at my departure I knew what I had come for and it was not for me to judge but his response told me that Jose also knew the end was near. Despite the inevitable outcome, there were more surprises to come.

A week after Christmas I received a telephone call to say that Jose had stabilised after my departure. This continued until several days before Christmas when he made a sudden and marked recovery. Two days before Christmas his doctors said Jose was in such good shape they felt quite confident for him, so he could go home.

Jose went home on Christmas Eve and spent a wonderful Christmas Day with his family. Like so many before, he was as he had always been, full of energy and so happy. Most important to Jose, was being at home playing with his grandchildren. The next day he was rushed to hospital and died soon after his arrival. Quite unexpectedly I had kept my promise to Jose, yet I shall never know how or why.

For some reason, for Jose and his family, his presence at home on that Christmas day was important, more than just being at home. It was not a whim or an idle wish when Jose replied, *"I want to be at home with my family for Christmas day."*

Gamblers win or lose by chance on the turn of a roulette wheel or the flip of a card but his was no gamble. No matter what the final result, whatever Jose's purpose of life was, it all seemed to have an inevitability drive about it.

My question was sudden, unexpected and totally intuitive. It was out of my mouth before I had time to think about it. Jose's instant reply must have penetrated deep in his inner intelligence. The answer was just as unexpectedly from his subconscious mind and there was an instant and long silence in the room. Everyone had good reason to freeze. At that time it was thought that Jose had at best a few days to live and Christmas was three weeks away. Tears instantly appeared in the eyes of those around him as everyone was fully aware of the reality so no one in that room believed it was possible.

Whatever the outcome, hidden somewhere in the detail there was and there always is an important reason for my participation. My visit to Jose was no different. Although things looked bleak, I had to understand that like Mark the racing car driver, it was alright that I did not understand at the time but to constantly be alert for the learning that will surely come.

Every patient is a master and every case history a profound teacher. My personal question was why Jose and not any of the other people who would die of cancer on that Christmas but for the sake of a support healer? In the beginning this question would trouble me. In answering it, the most important thing I remembered was that I am not the healer and I cannot be with all sick people. So, somewhere there are more reasons and answers to the questions "Why me and why so many are healed and why others do not make it?"

Though I was free to choose to answer the call for help or not, it was never really a choice of yes, no but rather how quickly I could be available. In retrospect it was like having an internal manager who picked the right event the right patient for the greatest success, failure or the next stage of my learning. Whichever, each has its own special story and brand of magic. As healers we all choose to be involved but experience has made it quite clear somewhere we are chosen for whom we will be involved with. I am not suggesting there is a God with his helpers sitting on a cloud checking their ledgers in order to manage this process. I am more comfortable with the possibility just as Albert Einstein believed it to be. There really maybe a field of energy and intelligence that links, connects and guides us all so we find the appropriate support when we need it,.

How does this work? Well I have no solid proof but asking patients how they found me, they invariably said something of the order that it was through a friend of a friend who knew someone who had heard of me. So telephone calls were made and the right information was passed down the line. Sometimes Ninian was that friend of a friend or occasionally people found themselves knocking on my door for no other reason than an intuitive feeling.

In the case of Mark the racing car driver, the analysis is reasonably straightforward because he lived for many years after. The proof was in the pudding to tell the tale. In the case of José how it worked is less easy to comprehend.

In battle conditions, soldiers have been known to be shot many times yet they have been so focused on their objective, they only fall and let go when they had achieved their goal. What we don't know is the whole story of Jose and his family. This is where we have to take a leap of a different trust that there was a really important reason for Jose to make that last brief recovery. In the great tapestry of life it could only be that Jose had something important to do and he needed a few extra days to complete his life and Christmas at home was that final and focused purpose or goal. While I saw him in hospital, underneath his struggle, at the end Jose didn't ask for a year or three or a long life he just asked for one special day.

Jose not only lives on in the spirit of this book he has also played his part in helping me to better understand the healing process. As I departed he already had a brighter light in his eyes. I saw it and dared to trust in another intuition.

In my experience of healing, very often the key act is simple, quick yet ultimately profound. Similar examples can be found throughout anyone's life. How often we search for a solution, then someone simply says; "what about............" with a moment's pause to make the thought pathway link, we say: "Of course, it's so simple but why on earth didn't I think of that before."

It is so important to remember that it's the mind and body/mind that we heal so the body can heal itself. In Jose's case this process seemed to have been a little more complex. His mind and body needed to be healed at least for a short while so that his mind could heal something else important to him and his family.

Whether searching for answers too difficult problems or overcoming an illness the key is to unlock the mental blockage that caused the problem in the first place. Healing comes in many forms, it doesn't have to be healing a blocked emotion or pain, it can just be unblocking a thinking pattern which is set in the wrong direction.

Healing can come from the most unlikely person or event. Everyone has the capacity to be that key for other people also under certain circumstances for themselves too. But understanding why or how the right person appears at the right moment can be difficult to comprehend mostly because we are never sure when the right time has arrived until afterwards.

Albert Einstein said: *"His greatest ideas came to him out of thin air and the soup of energy and intelligence that swirls around us all. He considered himself lucky to have found them before anyone else."*

Chapter 4

QUARRY WORKERS

One of Ninian's healing trips in Spain took me to the home of a woman in her early 50s. Immediately I saw her it was apparent by her body language that she was greatly troubled. A little later it became clear this woman was carrying the troubles and fears of her own world and that of her entire family on her shoulders. The problem was that her emotional stress was not only disturbing her health but also her family and neighbours had become exasperated by the constant torment. Worst of all, nobody could get her to talk about whatever was troubling her.

Christina would never share the details of her anguish with even the closest friend, her husband or family members. However, now the time was right and clearly time had played its role and Christina was ready to let go. The connection was that Christina was Ninian's secretary's aunt. Out of the blue Christina had asked her niece if she knew someone who could help her. Her niece knew about me so she asked Ninian to make the all important contact.

I sat down with Christina in her lounge. I had become used to the Spanish custom of the whole family joining in but this time I was slightly surprised when it seemed the entire street were invited or had they simply taken the right of open house to be part of this very unusual party.

In her stressed state Christina could tell me little more than was already known. Although she had asked for help the emotional blockage that prevented her releasing her anguish was still firmly in place. On reflection this behaviour appeared to be another form of the highly controlling "Want to but cannot," burnout syndrome. Although Christina was clearly in a state of overwhelming stress, I doubt she was in any degree of burnout. Listening to her I had the feeling of an enormous bottle of champagne being shaken by daily events. The pressure was mounting inside but the cork was securely wired in place leaving her mentally and physically distraught and under great emotional stress. I was clear that all I had to do was release the cork and then stand back. As others had done so Christina would inevitably do the rest of the healing herself.

The next stage was to move Christina to a deeply relaxed state. The process finally took three attempts at hypnotising her. Each time Christina would break down a little more of her resistance until eventually her eye lids began to flicker, she closed her eyes and for the first time in too many years she slipped into a calm, relaxed and peaceful sleep.

The marked lines and shadows of years of worry disappeared from her face, while her body became notably free of tension, as her hands with white knuckles turned pink again as she relaxed their grip on the chair arm rests. Keeping her in that state for several minutes was the second stage of the healing process. In the next few minutes Christina's breathing was deep and even. Her rapid eye movements beneath her closed eyelids indicated internally she was processing a lot of something.

In the room family and friends watched in anticipation and silence. I sensed a shifting energy as I made that now familiar mental connection with Christina's innate healing intelligence. No one else in the room noticed when a few moments later the subtle shift as the iron like hold on her emotional cork had been released. That almost imperceptible release is the telepathic signal that indicates the inner healer has done its work. It happens in a millisecond and is followed by a peaceful awareness that everything is now okay. There is nothing else to do but step back and watch what happens.

Christina looked around the room and remained silent for a minute or two. During those minutes the silence and tension grew perceptibly. It was a strange but electrically charged silence. Nonetheless it was clear something was happening but no one including myself knew what to expect. With a sudden gasp of air filling her lungs Christina exploded into a torrent of words bubbling and flowing with such a speed and force it was mesmerizing. This was Christina's moment to let go. Now she had finally popped her cork, so to speak, it was important for her to empty herself of everything that had stressed her for so long.

Christina unloaded nearly thirty years of daily fears for the safety of her husband and four sons, all of whom worked in the local marble quarry. She explained how the quarry had an appalling safety record, with serious accidents and occasional deaths from falling rock or when dynamiting the marble out of the rock face.

Christina had recounted practically each day of her life of fear for her family. It started from the day her husband and then one son after another went to work at the quarry. She mentally catalogued all accidents and every death at the quarry. When they happened each one was a new trauma of fear for the safety of her family. Now she had let go the accompanying emotions rose to the surface and the tears of healing bubbled up to ease away so much internal pain she had bottled up for so long.

Christina demonstrated the ability of the mind to remember and to create emotional blockages over a long period of time, also its capability to torment itself to the point of near self destruction. Christina had to face something very personal to reach the stage of asking for help. When she decided to let go was the first stage of restoring her inner healer but the pressure was so great she couldn't just sit down and explain everything. Something was blocked like a log jam in a river or a frozen sea way. Nothing can pass until the jam is cleared. In this case it was a little support from myself and a large showy explosion.

Chapter 5

TELEPATHY WITH A ROCK

John was the family leader, he had been the victim of a massive stroke. His family was lost without him. All their thoughts were how to bring the master home to carry on where he had left so abruptly. I arranged to meet the family at Romford Hospital, in the county of Essex on the northern outskirts of London. I was taken to the ward sister who had been notified that I was coming. She took me to where John was lying, she ushered the other members of the family out of the ward and returned to draw the curtains around John's bed to give us a little privacy.

Before she left us she gently whispered to me that John had had a massive stroke that normally would have killed any other person outright. She explained the doctors could not understand how it was possible he was still alive. I was told that John could see but could neither move nor could he close his eyes. He could not hear, speak or voluntarily move any part of his body. Immediately I got the message she was certain there was no way any healing miracle was going to happen that day. The ward sister gently let go of the curtain as she left the rock and me together.

Sitting on the edge of John's bed I turned to look into his eyes firmly fixed in an expressionless stare directly ahead. As the ward sister's words circulated in my mind, I looked into John's eyes and was all too aware of his family's expectations and the ward sister's subliminal message.

Once again like that of Mark and Jose, I wondered why I had been brought to this impossible situation. What could I hope to achieve? With so much brain damage, what was keeping John alive or why was he hanging onto the last thread of life so tenaciously?

There appeared to be nothing other than for me to help John to finally let go. Holding John's limp hand in mine I looked long and deep into his eyes, and asked that one important question, *"I have no idea what I can do to help you. What do you want me to do?* A few moments later I became aware that he wanted to speak to me.

Having experienced similar situations before, there was nothing to do but wait silently. When it came it was crystal clear. Telepathically I understood every word of John's story. He had been the undisputable leader, oracle and rock for his family and extended family. Nothing happened without first consulting John. His was the wisdom, and the last word. That is what he wanted and his family always had been used to, respected and had come to expect. Soon after his stroke, the family found themselves not only distraught but lost and floundering without their steersman, their guiding rudder, their rock of stability and protection.

At first I was surprised his family could be so selfish, so demanding, so unable to comprehend the gravity of the situation or the futility of their demands. Now aware of his story I began to understand who I had actually come to help.

John's last telepathic message was, *"please help them to understand and let me go. I cannot go back to what I was before; it is time they find their own leadership. I now realise that what I did was wrong, I have created this problem. Now I cannot leave until they are prepared to be the masters of their own lives."*

I parted the curtains and silently slipped away from John's bed, I knew what I had to do also knowing it would not be easy. The family of eight or nine members were in a group just a few yards from the ward entrance. Before I could say a word, in unison they said, *"when will he come home?"*

Momentarily I was shocked at the assumption that I could revive their leader so fast from an irreversible state. They had heard of my reputation and clearly they had great expectations. Also they had no idea of the enormous damage done to his brain even though the medical staff must have explained in detail what had happened to John and there was no going back.

Without warning that heavy weight of responsibility 'the restorer of life,' thumped onto my shoulders. I wanted to shout out that I wasn't God; I didn't have the power to recreate the miracle of life, and I was not even the real healer. But it wasn't the time for that and I knew it, so I prepared myself to be diplomatic, with discretion explaining the situation and doing what John had asked me to do.

When they came the words were hard, challenging without pity or compassion for the family. Telling them what had happened. Now for John it was the end and how they had to let him go. Pick up the reins of their own lives and learn to take responsibility for themselves. "Wow!" I thought, where did that come from?

Who was more shocked John's family or myself I'm not sure. With hardly a hesitation, two of the sons, like muscle bound rugby forwards, they both stepped towards me with but one clear spontaneous intention. As I prepared to defend myself from out of my mouth came the following words.

"I was your rock and am no more; if you love me let me go."

It was if the two sons instantly turned to stone in their forward rush while the rest of the family's protests were also stunned into silence. Though the words came out of my mouth, they were not my own voice. It was clear to see that the family knew precisely whose voice it was. In those few moments the group expression had turned from demand to shock, aggression and then straight into another emotional shock.

Then one of the daughters asked what they could do now. Still slightly shaken by what had happened, I quietly said, "Your father has asked that you find your own leadership so that he may be released to leave in peace."

Remarkably, for the first time, they understood the reality of the situation. Then I understood exactly why my message had been sufficiently brutal to shock them out of their refusal to accept what had happened to John.

A moment later the ward sister appeared through the door, addressing the family she said, *"I'm sorry to tell you that your father has passed away. He died just a few moments ago."*

I was no longer needed, my job was done, and John's family had many pressing things on their minds. This was my cue to discretely leave as the family reeled in those traumatic few minutes of absolute chaos. Coming for the first time to understand what they had to do, they had begun their own healing process. Once again the key act of healing was simple; short if not indeed the final part was a tad brutal. Though dramatic, the key was not just the shock to wake them up it was also to push the family out of their comfort zone, their familiar comfortable way of thinking. As usual the key to unlocking the healing process had to be exactly right to connect with all the inner feelings, emotions and defences of all those present in one penetrating hit. If I had planned it for a month I could not have imagined such a scenario.

When considering what activates spontaneous healing when a doctor says to a patient, I'm sorry but we have no more answers, you have a month to live. The shock of hearing those words will in some situations awaken something in the patient. Standing outside the hospital ward was a dramatic, stark, clinical environment, perhaps the most suitable place to wake up, in effect a cold shower of reality. Here the starkness of life and death, the bare walls, not even a simple seat for comfort. Here they stood with nothing but themselves. In that moment as they took their own leadership so John finally let go.

The question why me was patently clear? The answer was that I had the experience and the capability to telepathically communicate with the father and whilst planning to be diplomatic; my subconscious or inner intelligence knew exactly the right words to use and how to say them to maximum effect in the minimum amount of time.

We are mostly not aware of our inner body language even though it is shouting at us. Should we perchance acknowledge it does not mean we know how or what to do about it! The healing begins the moment we ask the right question.

Chapter 6

THE EMOTIONAL TRAP

Pedro and his wife had a beautiful daughter named Lisa. She was a great pride and joy to them. One day Lisa was on the pillion seat of her boyfriend's motorbike on a notoriously dangerous road in southern Spain. Despite the head-on collision at high speed with an oncoming van miraculously the boyfriend escaped with only minor injuries. He recovered from his superficial injuries to carry on doing what he had always done except he would never ride his motorbike again with Lisa.

Though Lisa was still alive and now at home she was bedridden. She could see, hear, move her body, arms and legs but couldn't speak or walk. The best she did was to make just a few noises some of which were recognisable words to her parents. I was marked by her eyes that betrayed her permanent and terrible fear.

Apart from remarkably few superficial wounds that had completely healed, the doctors considered Lisa had suffered a degree of brain damage. It was because of her apparent ability to understand her words that drove Pedro and his wife to make every effort to restore Lisa to normality. The hospital doctors had also encouraged them by saying anything was possible.

I had encountered similar cases but with little apparent immediate success. Despite this, I was always ready to search for the best way to participate with the patient's innate intelligence. I felt that if they had been brought to my attention then there was a good reason. Normally any healing session would be short, an hour perhaps, with the act of healing being relatively short, just a few minutes. Sometimes a healing session would be complete quite quickly such as Mark the racing car driver. In some cases it took more than one session. If there were no results by the third session, I considered for whatever the reasons, I was unable to be of any real further support. In some cases healing eventually happened as if spontaneously, which suggested to me the emotional blockage needed time to be cleared. Occasionally such as in Lisa's case where suspected brain damage was concerned, I allowed much longer even so I had to be mindful that brain damage may if that is indeed actually possible; take months or even many years to repair itself.

My initial contact with Lisa was devoted to finding how to make telepathic contact with her inner healer. After several attempts with no breakthrough, I diverted my effort to searching for something different or another way to access her damaged brain but still I had the intuitive feeling of being firmly if not forcibly kept out.

Finally the time came for me to return to England, there was no change in Lisa, there was no telepathic communication or intuitive guidance. Frustratingly there was a strong feeling that my trip had been important though I could see no evidence of it so I put the feeling down to wishful thinking. I wondered what had gone wrong or what had I missed. This time the question "why me" had a whole new meaning. Why had those communication connections involved me and thus, why had I failed? This was not simply a mistake to learn something from, it was more profound than that. What could I learn from this? This was not one of Ninian's contacts so why had Pedro and his wife heard about me? Why should they and Lisa suffer and the boyfriend get off scot-free? He had not even gone to visit Lisa. None of this conformed to other cases, therefore I felt I had missed or overlooked something important or I had accidentally interfered.

I have discussed this case with many people among them a number of healers and yes, they all offered their sympathetic reasons and answers to those questions.

"*God has a mission for you and it's not for you to understand these things or question them,*" was again the favourite or typical comment. For me this answer is fickle and plagued with irresponsible ignorance that leads so many people to trust their lives to inadequate superstitious beliefs and false faith in something they have little or no understand of.

I needed to find reliable answers to my questions. I could not accept the idea that God is responsible for everything while we are just puppets. We either take responsibility for our lives or we live like automaton sheep. I may be involved in something quite out of the ordinary and traditionally steeped in superstition but I had no truck with blind faith, apathy and ignorance allowing myself to be snagged on the bramble thorns of hollow idles of false and foolish beliefs.

Intuitively I felt I had done what was required but I had no way of knowing what I had done. So was this awareness of doing the right thing actually intuition or was it indeed wishful thinking or could it be an ego saving exercise. The answers were there, it was a matter of careful observation, detailed analysis with a lot of patience to learn the truth and hopefully the whole truth.

While pondering on all these questions, I suddenly spotted a significant difference in this attempted support healing. This was related to by conclusion that when I made telepathic contact with the patient's innate healing intelligence, in return I received telepathic guidance as to precisely what I had to do. In Lisa's case I made the telepathic contact but there was no telepathic or intuitive feedback. This explained the sensation I had of deliberately being shut out. Then I remembered the look of a terrible fear in Lisa's eyes.

I had to keep reminding myself that I am not the healer only the key. Lisa had apparently sustained brain damage but was there something different about this case. Dr Deepak Chopra quotes a case in his book Quantum Healing of a similar road accident and brain damage, yet the young man recovered fully.

Despite her parent's wishes that I keep on trying I could not account for the feeling Lisa was resisting and I was sensing her resistance by the feeling of an impenetrable closed door. It was clear the more I was to understand healing, the more I had to understand the psychology even the paradoxes of the body/mind, the inner healer and subconscious or inner intelligence. Therefore, it was equally important to understand why sometimes the key and the healing processes do not appear to work.

My only hope is that this is somehow true. My hope is in an incredibly subtle and gentle way Lisa's innate healing intelligence gradually entices her survival and self protection system intelligence buried in its deep safety cave, to let go of the fear and come out into the light. It is with this inner guidance that I began to make some reasonable understanding that after my initial efforts I was lured into interfering by trying to get Lisa to respond. Certainly accidents like Lisa's can leave people permanently in a cabbage like state. There are however numerous cases of complete recovery despite the doctors and surgeons worst prognosis. Dr. Weil refers to such cases in his book 'Spontaneous Healing.' Earlier I referred to a man who suffered severe concussion and brain damage. He woke up to find he had rewired his brain to the degree that without one lesson he was not only supremely competent at playing the piano, he was constantly composing beautiful melodies as he played.

My healing gift and developed skills depended greatly on feelings and refined intuitive awareness intelligence. In this work, feelings like intuition and telepathy are most important especially when there is no means of communicating through speech. I recognise as there was no response from Lisa, my desire to be seen to achieve something undoubtedly got in the way of intuitive intelligence. In short I began to realise that was how I had tricked myself into the emotional trap of interfering.

I began a logical analysis and to see my effort as my failure. Had it merely been an ego trip gone wrong, and frankly a waste of time and money? Overriding this negative logic and every emotion or feelings, there was always that sense that Lisa could recover if she wanted to.

After many years of studying thought patterns I realised that those feelings of resistance were an important clue as to what had happened in Lisa's mind. Lisa was alive and her bodily functions worked normally. This meant that her inner intelligence and inner healer were also functioning at least at the level of repairing and maintaining the body structure and basic maintenance. This raised the question if the inner healing intelligence has the capability to heal, rebuild and restore internal functions, why does it not restore all brain and emotional functions too.

I was reminded of an horrific accident where a car driver had been distracted and ran into the back of a builders truck. A scaffold pole penetrated his skull and he survived to tell the tale. In another case a construction worker fell onto upstanding concrete reinforcing bars. One bar passed through his skull and others through his body but he recovered fully. For these reasons I suspect part of the answer, is Lisa had chosen to stay precisely where she was and well out of any future harm's way.

The fact she could not or would not talk or walk may be a key to protecting herself from ever doing the same thing again. Many years later after my experience of burnout and the "Want to but cannot or will not syndrome," I wondered if after the accident she had suffered her own nightmare burnout.

In six words it is "thinking I knew what was best." This was not because Lisa was a pretty young woman and the apple of her father's eye, or that I had travelled a long way to do a job and I had my own expectations to perform well. Knowingly or unknowingly, I came to realise how I stepped into the emotional trap because of the injustice. Lisa was innocent of responsibility for her condition. For the first time, I allowed myself to be caught up in my feelings that she deserved to live her life to the full. To compound this I ignored my awareness of her resistance and poured my energy and resources into solving the problem. Not surprisingly, the more I did this Lisa's resistance responded by holding ever more strongly to her own resolve. Now I had confirmation that it is pointless the healer thinking they know what to do or what is right for the patient. This is just as it is futile to impose healing on anyone and certainly not someone who does not want it.

Some time later a boy of ten years old and severely mentally retarded was brought to me by an acquaintance of many years. I had few expectations but agreed to do what I could. Intuitively I felt the boy would be inhibited by his parents so I chose to work on him in a separate room without their presence. The doors were left open wide so all was within ear shot but just out of sight. Curiosity is itself a curious thing, thus so, the parents were at liberty to peek around the corner if they wished. The boy spent his time giggling throughout my efforts to make telepathic contact with his subconscious mind. I hoped any change in this behaviour might indicate a change was happening. After several sessions there was no change and the parents stopped the healing. The look of aggression in the father's eyes at that time spoke of deep resentment. The occasional times I bumped into him indicated his son had not improved. I have no real idea what may have been going on in the father's traumatised mind, though I suspect he had no good words for me despite my efforts to do what I could. This case was a brain problem from birth and my intuitive feelings were that little good result would be achieved. It all shows there are limitations to even the greatest gift or understanding of how to activate spontaneous healing. I am not even sure the boy understood what was happening. If he did not understand there was anything wrong with him, he had no reason to want healing. If there was a fundamental lacking of conscious awareness, then my efforts were pointless and therefore irrelevant.

The answer and learning for all healing therapists no matter what their speciality, is to always respect intuition and avoid doing things for friends, acquaintances or for old time sake, when it is clear a positive outcome is bleak to say the best. Finally, if it amounts to interfering as this case did, then healing of this nature has no chance.

In Lisa's case in order to reduce travel costs and complex timetable connections I had committed myself to several days so I stayed the course. Half way through I believed Lisa would remain as she was until she had accepted to learn something about herself. There are stark similarities with the case of Mark the racing driver, where an inner intelligence refused to let go and locked up his muscles as if to say; *"You will stay like this until you have learnt to accept yourself as you are and not to drive racing cars anymore as an escape."*

In Lisa's case I can imagine her not wanting to put herself at risk again was a reverse of Mark's syndrome. Even so intuitively I felt there was something else at work. When I got to meet Mark it was apparent that he had already accepted what he had to learn, though may be he had not quite let go because of the problem of the macho image. Like Mark, and in chapter 8, the Spanish Doctor had also learnt something important that allowed him to accept healing from a non orthodox medical healer.

It is necessary to consider the body/mind – subconscious mind also Lisa's conscious will. At this point I am reminded of the minds survival and self protection intelligence. This evolves from the subconscious mind, and driven by emotional intelligence, it can be ferociously powerful. Her actual thought processes might be difficult to discover if indeed many years later she is capable or willing to tell her story. I am reminded of the expression "you may lead a horse to water but you cannot make it drink."

At the time and for a long time after it had not occurred to me that no one had consulted Lisa for obvious reasons. The assumption was that what her parents wanted is what Lisa wanted and they were doing the right thing. Does anyone ever consider what is happening in the mind at the conscious and subconscious level of a terrible and traumatic accident victim even if they escape unscathed physically?

I had attended NLP and life coaching courses where I learnt the theory of mind filters, mental barriers and other emotional blocking devices. Learning about these things is quite different to experiencing them at work in other people. It has been cases like Lisa's that have helped me to understand these delicate filters have absolute control over many centres of intelligence and habitual behaviours of the mind. This certainly includes survival and self protection intelligence and the inner healer, especially in the case of suffering dramatic traumas.

Just put yourself in the inner trauma Lisa must have experienced. You are on the back of a motorbike travelling at high speed. You may be anxious but you are young and enjoying life. The driver you have your loving arms so tightly wrapped around suddenly pulls out to overtake in a spontaneous moment of opportunity. You see the oncoming van suddenly pull out in front of you and hear the screeching of tyres milliseconds before you feel that initial body crunching impact as the motor bike slams into the oncoming van. With the air punched out of your lungs and flung like a rag doll into the air, the conscious trauma realisation must be catastrophic. But this tale is not yet finished because there is no understanding of what is happening in the subconscious mind. After the first impact you are aware of not being able to breathe as you fly over the oncoming van. At the same moment you are conscious of your helpless plight and the truck following behind the first van. Like a terrible torture, first having the air punched out of your lungs and then flung into the air, now you are faced with the next mind shattering part of the nightmare. This is the final impact as you crash through the truck's glass windscreen. That is the moment when you lose consciousness. Yet in that state your subconscious intelligence is aware of what is happening to you.

It is hard to truly visualise let alone understand what Lisa experienced in those moments which probably to her seemed like an eternity. How many times daily does she relive those horrendous images with the memory of wrenching pain tearing through her body and mind? Could it be that she lives one constant recycling time warp replaying the horror over and over again, day after day, night after night? If this is the case it is hardly surprising that I noticed she had a permanent look of a terrible fear in her eyes.

In their book "Seven Life Lessons of Chaos" John Briggs and F. David Peat explain how the chaos theory keeps us alive. Layer upon layer upon layer of chaos driven feedback loops circulate, constantly realigning our life forces to maintain an air of order we call a state of ease and good health.

In the space of a few seconds Lisa had entered an infernal chaos far beyond the norm that has possibly looped around and around with little or no chance of restoring what we would consider to be a new direction, a new phase for her growth and evolution. But strangely that is possibly exactly what has happened. Lisa might easily have died. Somewhere in her internal survival system intelligence she decided to live. I do believe the fighting and resisting of external healing, is evidence that she chose to live but is frightened to live for the fear of all that stuff happening again. Is she still whirling around in her own extremely personal chaotic tumbling nightmare while constantly erecting protective walls to guard her from all that she perceives a terrible outside world could do to her again only to see those disintegrate as that truck windscreen had done.

Only when she finds the confidence to put the pieces of her jig-saw puzzle of that chaos into place, will she find the courage to change her present state. Unwittingly, her mother and father, myself and maybe many others caught up in her story are all linked into the same chaos that will lead us to something else. It is fruitless to fight it. Our only hope is to immerse ourselves in it then go with the flow of energy that brought us all together and then find what learning we can from the entire experience that we may better understand others who experience such a trauma.

Though I generally dislike this type of reasoning because it speaks with a certain authority about souls that in truth we have no proof of, thus it is all beliefs and theory presented as something more factual than anyone has a right to impose. Nonetheless, for all of us and that now means you. As you read this story, you may think Lisa's story will be quickly forgotten. Hopefully it will stay with you even if you think it is just another story of yet another road accident.

Lisa was out of another mould and she may have been too young and inexperienced to know she had options or opportunities other than the plight she is now in. It may be all supposition but could have Lisa gone with the flow as her boyfriend apparently did and come out of a nasty accident practically unscathed other than some haunting memories and being a little wiser after the event.

Did she choose to grab the iron bar of self imprisonment in front of her part way down that tunnel of chaos during and immediately after the accident? Is that what has kept her hanging in suspension and unable to let go? How often can, what may seem to be safe solutions, actually prove to be throwing ourselves from the frying pan into the fire? In this scenario, can anyone not wonder that her inner survival and self protection intelligence would want to do anything other than retreat into the safety of her inner mind and slam the door shut on the outside world? Bolted and secure until she feels safe to emerge, she reels in that chaos memory of physical and emotional pain, fear and shock. Perhaps as the case of Mark, her inner emotional intelligence was screaming over and over, "do not ever do that to me again." The greatest danger is in her turning a survival strategy into a way of life, in, which case there is no way out.

Had her parents interfered prematurely and did I arrive too early to do what I had done for Mark? Will a young handsome healer Prince arrive at the perfect moment to give this sleeping beauty a helping hand to release her from her own prison tower when she is ready, or will what I did without knowing accelerate the process so she naturally breaks out under her own steam?

Dr. Andrew Weil, M.D. says in his book 'Spontaneous Healing'-
"But when I look at the role of emotions in facilitating spontaneous healing, I think it may be more useful to encourage sick people to cultivate passion. I have mentioned healing responses that occur after falling in love or expressing anger. Whether the emotion felt is positive or negative seems not to matter; rather it is the intensity of the feeling that gives it power to affect body function. More than negative feelings, apathy may be the major emotional obstacle to spontaneous healing."

After such an ordeal what remotest of wish could anyone have to venture out into the world again? We must remember this is a trauma beyond our comprehension. There is no means of knowing how Lisa processes her own chaos. If she needed to slam the door on her future life, we have no option but to respect that. When someone is in this state, like the story of the wife and mother in the case history of "Quarry workers," only when a person is ready inside, will they open the door to outside help to be released from their self made emotional prison.

Thus in Lisa's case, it may just be that my feeling of her resistance and being shut out was because she simply felt she was not yet ready to come out to play in the sunshine once again.

Chapter 7

ALONE AND DESPERATE

Judy was suffering badly with stomach cancer. She ran the gauntlet of surgery, chemotherapy, radiation treatment plus some fairly devastating medications. Eventually her doctor told her the treatment had failed, indeed the tumour had spread throughout her body and was growing at an alarming rate. She had just a few weeks to live, sort out her life and try to tie up the loose ends. Judy contacted me through a friend who had heard of my support healing.

Judy was a single parent with a young son. Her husband had been fit and an active sportsman. Just a year before Judy's cancer, in a traumatic few months her husband had been taken by the same cancer. Judy, already traumatised by the loss of her husband had no other family so she was now frantic about her son's future.

Judy was a tall elegant woman but the stress and trauma that was now her life was clearly written in her posture, her words, and marked on her face and in her eyes. Her inner executioner was her constant companion demanding that the inevitable shall happen and soon. This courageous woman who had been given notice of her death had chosen to turn into a tornado of panic for one reason only that of protecting her son's future. The only way I can describe Judy's behaviour, is blind panic laced with a deadly cocktail of fear. There is nothing so strong as a mother's defence of her offspring.

The chemotherapy and radiation treatments had already depleted her immune system. Now her powerful emotions were skyrocketing her stress levels thus causing her body to be flooded with cortisol and other damaging hormones that were destroying her immune system even further. The result was that with no defences, her cancer was ravaging her body unhindered.

I was struck by her incredible capacity to find the energy she needed to keep going when others only half as ill would be confined to their bed. I felt I could do no more than accept that this time I really had no answers and was staring at defeat unless I came up with a real copper bottomed; gold plated support healing that did whatever it did to get her back on track.

At this time I had not fully worked out the fine detail of the crucial element of my support healing that later proved to be the real key. I have since concluded that as her immune and innate healing systems were so depleted due to the medical treatment, there was nothing left. The former power of her innate healing intelligence had no more fight to effect healing from the inside. Even if I had evolved that far, I believe her emotional panic was powerful enough to block anything my support healing was capable of. Although at that time a fledging theory that I was the support act not the real healer, at the very least I understood I must make that telepathic link to gain access to her innate healing intelligence and gain its consent to work with me. Ultimately when her inner healing intelligence is broken so it cannot respond, then there is truly no hope. The inability to do this drew me into wanting to help her with everything I knew and thought could be helpful. Of course at this point I had crossed that red line of not interfering but in this case it made no difference.

While these issues are of interest and important, if I had the real power of healing in me, the force of my terrifying focus would have without any doubt blasted any cancer cells into oblivion. I believe this does at least give a degree of credence to the conclusion that as a support healer, much like any doctor or surgeon, I was not the real healer. I was only capable of alerting and thus enabling a patient's inner healing intelligence to do its own work.

In this situation I wondered how could interfering do anything so wrong? Well, as my understanding of the sensitivity of the innate healing intelligence grew, I realised that wrong is wrong no matter what colour or reason it comes packed in. Wrong is wrong because it is inevitably tied to the emotional trap of wanting to be the healer, wanting to play God and supercharge the core spark of life. Beyond these important factors, any level of interference simply gets in the way of the patient's innate healer. The inevitable ending was writ large on the wall of her life as her innate healer had been destroyed by the cancer treatment. Thus so, I concluded anything I did to help at that stage could at least do no more harm.

In our complex world of boundaries, beliefs, social and business regulations and judicial laws, we understand that it all works by a process of bending with the wind, going with the flow and adaptations to suit the situation. These rules and laws are intended to evolve or change in line with social needs. In understanding the nuances of brain/mind intelligence centres, DNA programs and support healing, I have come to accept how the body's innate centres of intelligence are another universe that does not appear to have that capacity to make adjustments to long standing genetic programs. This is why we have doctors, hospitals and support healers. Analysing so many case histories, my conclusion is that subconscious intelligence and therefore innate healing intelligence work by a very special set of rules that I have yet to understand or master.

One reason for this is because they are DNA pre-installed programs; they have no capability to adjust to sentiments. Yes they can become blocked or in part switched off by traumatic events but they cannot automatically reprogram themselves at the drop of a hat.

DNA programs of information and intelligence can be changed relatively quickly. Now there is the possibility these developments can help healing in a very special way. Unfortunately, when working with Judy my awareness and expertise in this field was some way in my future. Thirty years later I now work with new performance programs designed to change events that can be inserted in a matter of seconds. What the old fashioned healers were doing believing they were the healer was effectively trying to change old programs wilfully simply by their faith. Now that is possible, not by faith healers and wishful thinking but by neuroscience and carefully designed performance programs. This is not interfering but intervening in a positive and dynamic way. This is essentially what sports-mind performance coaches do for high sports performance coaching. Now it is easier and quicker to shut down old and limiting programs by deactivating them. Alternatively parking them in a virtual mind siding while replacing them with purpose designed new behaviour programs. In short, this is done by creating completely new behaviour programs by radically changing the way we think and behave within subconscious mind thinking.

In the past I had experienced many staggeringly successful healing cases, these were proof positive for me that I had been doing something right. Judy's is another case that played an important part in me better understanding the process of spontaneous healing having to come from inside the patient and not something done to them from the outside. This is evident in the fact surgeons from the outside had done all they were capable of. That was all mechanical or plumbing detail focused on only the cancer cells. That had ignored her catastrophic emotional trauma of losing her husband and then fighting for her own life and to be with her son.

The power of her trauma had the emotional capability to block the best the surgeons could offer in their effort to help. What she could not grasp was in fighting like a lion, she was feeding her trauma stress while also blocking what was left of her innate healing system.

As Judy explained the loss of her husband, the shock trauma of his death to her was frighteningly clear to perceive. Like a massive earthquake and the shifting tectonic plates of her inner world, they sent a gigantic tsunami shock wave through her inner balance. Judy's mind was like a spacial black hole; it swallowed everything in its path in her search for a way to stop the cancer and save her son. In the end, it seems that level of panic is so powerful that it has nowhere to go but self-destruct its own survival intelligence systems and in Judy's case another life has unnecessarily gone prematurely.

We all understand that panic is not a good idea in any event. Panic is unpredictable; it destroys reason and balance as it scatters its forces in all directions with little return. It snatches with futility at straws for salvation. Success in the teeth of chaos even at lightning speed is a careful and steady process to keeping the flow of energy focused and under control to get it where it really needs to be. Mostly when getting this right in the midst of chaos it mainly works by intuitive intelligence. Without knowledge of how the mind works it is not easy to link with our intuitive or telepathic intelligence.

The case of the Spanish doctor is the same cancer condition and scenario of secondary tumours but a totally different mindset of an uncanny calmness. Certainly he had a large and close family so he did not have the same panic stress to protect a son. Also due to his calmness he was capable of willingly changing a lifelong held belief that all spiritual or faith healers were fakes. From all he later told me, I can only believe that it was in listening to his intuitive intelligence that enabled him to ask for my support. This was dramatically different than Judy's case, as she was throwing herself, one at a time at any and every alternative healing option she heard of.

Dr Deepak Chopra talks about cancer as cellular programming that has lost its way so it becomes undirected, permanently chaotic and finally self destructive. Perhaps you recognise the same thinking strategy pattern that led Jim the businessman to destroy his own company believing he was doing everything to save it. Likewise, Judy's out of control thinking was feeding her out of control cancer with ever more momentum. I often wondered what more could be done without interfering in the need to turn the clock back.

Chapter 8

A SPANISH DOCTOR

Ninian was on the telephone asking if I would help a doctor in Spain. He had been through chemotherapy, operations and all the treatment Spanish hospitals could offer. Now he only had two weeks to live. I thought it was leaving such an important thing a little late but even so I was on the first available flight to Malaga. After a short relaxed discussion the doctor calmly lay down on a bed. I sensed a state of tension in him so avoided hypnosis, instead relying on helping him enter a gentle state of relaxation. Intuitively I felt he was ready so held my hands one or two inches above his stomach. With no preconceived ideas of what I should do other than making the important telepathic link, I simply responded to the moment and guidance of the doctor's innate healing intelligence.

The doctor's eyes were closed, he breathed gently, there was an air of peaceful relaxation and he appeared like a child in a deep untroubled, untouchable sleep. The process of healing took no more than five or six minutes, though with the introductions and discussion afterwards about 30 minutes in all.

I revived the doctor when I felt there was no more to be done. After a few moments of silence he opened his eyes, and then he said that he felt as if a laser beam of intense light had burnt his cancer. Two weeks after our meeting, I had a call from Ninian to say the doctor was back at work, and there was no trace of the cancer.

A little over a year and a half later, returning home from a skiing holiday late one Sunday evening, I checked my answer phone. There was an urgent call asking for my help. The doctor had suffered a massive heart attack. He was in a military hospital near Gibraltar. Ninian had been trying to contact me every day. The doctor was hanging onto life by a thread but insisting to see and talk to me.

I caught the next available flight to Gibraltar. I entered the hospital under the guise of his English lawyer, which his family knew his privacy would be respected with no interruptions. On one side of a large private room were members of his family about twelve people in all. From their presence it was clear to me how serious the doctor's condition really was. I had experienced this same behaviour in Spanish families whatever the problem but this time the atmosphere was quite different. We greeted each other and then I sat down but the doctor was impatient and launched immediately into everything he needed to unload and for which he had hung onto life for two weeks to tell me. Later I made the connection with the same reserves of a dwindling life spark as Jose had shown in beating all the odds so he could be at home with his family on that Christmas day.

Although in an intense emotional state, he explained that he knew he was dying but could not go before telling me what happened after our first meeting and healing. He recounted how the immediate and rapid recovery and disappearance of his cancer had been incredible at the same time it caused him serious emotional unrest and soul searching. He explained how throughout his career as a doctor, he had been a scientist relying on medical fact. He had been vehemently against faith or spiritual, in fact any form of alternative healing; due to his conviction it was all fraudulent. Then when he was on the threshold of death, when medical science had no more solutions, what he had rejected for so long and so aggressively had literally come out of the blue to hand him back his life.

He referred to what I did as spiritual healing. I felt this was not the time for explaining that was not quite what I believed. Could that have made the difference to save his life a second time even though at that moment, I did not have the full knowledge and understanding as I have today? He explained his internal confusion of medical science and his firsthand experience of what I had done with healing and how that grew into an enormous emotional trauma of conscience. This consumed his daily thoughts while also reflecting on his entire life and medical career. He explained how he realised he was building an enormous stress, which had likely brought about his heart attack.

I had no time to convince him of the neuroscience of spontaneous healing; it would have simply been too long and demanding in his state. Also I was depending on Ninian as interpreter, so if the doctor, Ninian or both did not understand what I was talking about in terms of neuroscience, it could have turned into an enormous and stressful mess. These were his last words. I was there to listen to the doctor not argue with him or press my case. Thus I was forced to perhaps wrongly accept the doctor believing my support healing as of a spiritual nature. He was now convinced all his professional life he had been wrong about healing. Apparently he had now acknowledged alternative or spiritual healing did have a place just as his orthodox medical training and profession had. Despite this he had a great concern because I was his only experience and that meant to him; there could still be many charlatans on the streets. What troubled him so much was the fact he did not understand how the healing worked. Further troubling to him was the fact I did not appear to be at all religious or of any spiritual inclination.

As a doctor these facts represented an irrational, unreliable contradiction of everything he understood and relied on. He didn't know anymore what he could trust in or of what was solid or dependable to sustain his reason to be a doctor and thus a worthy member of the medical profession.

The doctor spoke for what seemed more than an hour. At one time his emotion was so great he had a seizure. I held him in my arms for several minutes, the only thing I could do. Then he recovered and though then very weak, he continued with what he needed so desperately to share with me. His entire discourse amounted to an analysis of what he experienced during the healing, its simplicity and short duration also his attempts to rationalise medical science with what he experienced during the healing. Interestingly one of his conclusions was the question of intrinsic values and emotional energy, better referred to today as emotional intelligence. When he had finished he was clearly hovering on the edge of life and death. Undoubtedly these were his last moments for his family to be close to him. Ninian took me to a house half an hour's drive from the hospital. Just as we arrived the telephone rang, the message was passed to Ninian to say the doctor had died peacefully a few minutes earlier.

Of all the doctor told me, it was the detail of his feelings and confusion marked by one important underlying message that stood out. Although it was clear he only had a few days to live, he was aware his mind was calm and stable. During the following months because he could not find the answers or because he could not accept the answers his mind turned to uncontrollable chaos. A pattern was forming of a combination of high stress, emotional chaos and sustained panic being connected to cancer and heart attacks.

The Spanish doctor eventually died due to a massive heart attack. No doubt his heart was weakened by his cancer chemotherapy treatment and further weakened by massive amounts of cortisol due to his new found confusion and emotional chaos.

My explanation of the doctor's awareness of a laser beam burning the cancer was perception alone. This is likely the work of his inner healing intelligence. I can only guess as to the reason for this being an indicator of a technology that he would understand. Therefore, as we all experience dreams, intuition or insights, his innate healing intelligence gave his conscious mind something he could easily and quickly associate with.

As Ninian had clearly made a strong argument for why his friend should follow his advice, I believe the doctor persuaded himself - why not test it now, what is there to lose. All credit to him for making the mental shift and so absolutely accepting the unthinkable and the unknown so willingly. The Spanish doctor's capacity to traumatise his mind over the healing experience but not be traumatised by his cancer was clear in all he desperately needed to share with me in his dying minutes.

I accept the concept of spirituality is a complex subject but please let this be a lesson to us all to be sure not to get spirituality, faith and spontaneous healing mixed up with the innate healing system and emotional intelligence; in one irrational mess.

There is no doubt that we are all our greatest healer or the cause of our worst suffering or illness. We have the choice but for the desire to know it, understand it, use it or change it.

One lesson I took from this case is that anyone going through a dramatic healing, will inevitably have a need for continued support to avoid crashing into emotional chaos.

Mahatma Ghandi said of succeeding,

"You must be the change that you want to see in your own world."

Chapter 9

CONNECTING A WRIST

George was a senior aircraft salesman in his mid fifties. Some years earlier he had been involved in a serious accident where he almost lost his right hand. Surgeons saved his hand but the technology to do more at that time had not yet been developed so the nerves were permanently severed leaving him with no feeling or practical use of that hand. About two years later new surgical advancement became available. George was contacted and told if he wished he could have an operation to rejoin his severed nerves.

When I met George it was about two years after the nerves running through his wrist had been reconnected. His face had that greyed, strained look typical of people enduring long term pain and suffering. He explained how the operation itself was carried out successfully. Unfortunately, afterwards he had the sensation his hand was permanently in boiling water. First the doctors had given him powerful pain killers, then later he was fitted with a gadget strapped to the palm of his hand. He explained how the new gismo vibrates at a specific frequency to counter the nerve signal chaos that created the burning sensation. This helped but only partially.

I sat in front of George holding his wrist for a few moments. The telepathic handshake was working but in an extraordinary way. This time, I was aware of watching a mental video of a telephone engineer joining two huge cables, each with thousands of coloured wires. The problem was that most of the wires had been cross linked. In the telephone exchange (George's brain) there was total pandemonium as most nerve signals were being routed to the wrong addresses.

I explained to George what I had just experienced, he said, *"yes it's exactly like that, that's how the surgeons explained what they suspected was causing the burning sensation and the gadget was designed to mask the chaos."*

Here again was a completely new experience for me. I really had no idea how I was able to help his innate healing system reroute the messaging from nerves that were physically rejoined incorrectly. Even so, sticking to my strategy of no interference, and the patient's innate healing intelligence knowing best, I was game to do whatever his inner healing intelligence needed. I realised my feelings and thoughts were getting so close to interfering due to the apparent impossibility of this project. What troubled me was a two pronged potential torpedo to the healing. First, this was so unusual, I had no idea how his innate healing intelligence could possibly have a game plan. Second was the fact of me simply having this limiting thought could so easily get in the way of a successful outcome.

I found it necessary to re-centre myself with no expectations and no preconceived ideas of what is or is not possible. Now I was open to whatever George's innate healer knew could work and that meant anything was possible. I had already come to accept that healing worked in the most unlikely situations so this was a great opportunity to expand my knowledge.

Again I relied on my intuition to guide me in the healing process and a few minutes later George put his head back opened his eyes and made that familiar smile of coming out of a hypnotic trance. When fully conscious he became aware of his hand. His eyes opened wide in amazement. Some colour had already returned to his face also much of the stress lines were gone. Unbelievably he looked at his hand and said, *"it feels so much better."*

I met George some months later when we had another session. After the first healing some of the pain had gradually returned, nonetheless he assured me the support healing had led to a great improvement. Following the second healing there was again a notable improvement but not total healing.

So much we know about the brain and mind today was not yet fully in the public domain in those days. Some months later I had another call from George. Although he still had a slight hot sensation in his hand, he was not always conscious of the sensation, so he felt it was gradually correcting itself. I didn't hear from him again therefore concluded his inner healer continued to perform its own magic otherwise the remaining warm sensation was of no great consequence.

Today neuroscientists would likely explain that his brain had learnt to reroute or rewire most of the nerve signals so the nerve ending in his hand and wrist connected with the appropriate sensory intelligence within his brain. This procedure has been recorded in brain research when people survive brain damage where they lost memory or specific capabilities. Today the medical healing process includes training to help the person create new thinking pathways using parts of the brain not normally used in that way. In some ways this is similar to wide band mobile telephone signals. The wider you make the band or pathway, the more information can pass through and faster. Another more familiar metaphor is the case of those who lose their sight so the brain re-routes sight sensitivity to new developments of advanced hearing capability and other sensory awareness such as a greater command of intuitive intelligence.

In a recent case reported during 2016 a man lost his sight after receiving a bang on his head. Thirty five years later he recovered his sight after a similar bang to his head. This indicates how nothing was broken but even a small trauma like banging ones head can switch senses on and off. A young woman in Afghanistan receives a bullet in the head and survives to become a women's and children's' rights advocate. A famous racing driver has a fall while skiing. He is wearing a helmet but still the impact against a rock leaves him severely disabled. Clearly the defining lines of brain function relative to injury are complex.

During August 2016 a story as mentioned earlier that broke internationally was about a number of paralysed Brazilian men who recovered a degree of lower body feeling after being fitted with an exoskeleton to give them back the ability to walk again. During ten months of training the scientists found the men's brains were automatically re-routing nerve messaging through surface muscle tissue, thus bypassing their damaged spinal cords. My immediate question was why did those men need exoskeletons to trigger this unusual process. What is if any, the connection between the external support of an exoskeleton and my external support healing to cause similar processes to happen.

Therefore my principle question concerning George's accident is this. Why over two years of treatment after George's operation to reconnect the nerves in his wrist, didn't his brain correct the nerve signal alignment automatically? In answering this I would suggest this following scenario to both cases. I accept it is completely hypothetical though based on my healing and research experience relative to emotional intelligence.

We cannot know what happened in George's conscious thoughts and certainly can never know what happened in the subconscious mind at the time of the accident and following trauma. Neither can we know of or understand what the emotional and survival effect was to his innate healing intelligence. The fact of his hand being severed followed by it being stitched back on but having no usability, would surely be an ongoing trauma to him. At the very least this would be manifested in his daily visual reminder of the accident and the first shock of losing his hand. Then two years later having the unexpected operation of his nerves being rejoined to return feeling and control to his hand, would have surely had considerable additional immediate emotional ramifications and longer term consequences of possibly a fear of it ultimately going wrong.

This case is similar in many ways to Mark's, the Spanish doctor's and Lisa's case, i.e. each case is linked to a traumatic accident or belief or value situation. In Marks case there was a shock trauma caused at the time of the accident and perhaps compounded over the months afterwards. This was as his conscious mind reminded itself every time it saw, felt or relived those devastating moments of his accident with the consequent results. At the time of George's accident, the thought of losing his right hand; although the surgeons were able to save it must have emotionally haunted him constantly.

I know that when reminded of near accidents or silly things I have done in the past, how I can shiver at the very thought of a near miss regardless of the fact that nothing untoward actually happened. For some reason emotional intelligence thought and connected imagination of what could have happened has a stronger impact on our brain, mind and memories than what actually happened, albeit what did happen may be troubling.

In the beginning George still had his hand, this was certainly a blessing but not to be able to use it would have been a considerable frustration and possibly a severe embarrassment. Although he had regained considerable use of the hand after the second operation to connect his severed nerves, he told me of his depression in wondering if the endless pain was really worthwhile.

Therefore, my support healing may have started George's emotional process of disconnecting those shock and emotional barriers. The more his trauma emotion was weakened, the less he was consciously aware of his hand and the memory of the accident. If it is possible, the self healing blockage was the trauma memory. As the trauma is healed the inner healer is released to do what it has evolved to do in its inimitable way.

If so, it seems the mind could not or would not automatically activate its own healing capabilities until George had recognised something about the accident or the trauma. Was the blockage to natural healing that he needed to accept or resolve his inevitable fears in order to allow the inner healing to begin its work?

By this stage of my healing progression I had begun to adopt more coaching methods to support my patients in getting to the underlying problem. This may seem to be a contradiction of what I said about non-interference from the healer and there being no need for the healer to know or understand what has happened or why. However, first the coaching is mainly to move the patient's thinking out of a victim state or some other negatively driven thinking process. Second, the important leaning processes are primarily for the patient and not for the healer.

Coaching is exceedingly good at helping the patient get to understand, accept and overcome or heal their own fear or trauma. Nonetheless; in this case as in many; it has not been possible to recognise exactly what part of the healing process had touched the vital link that released George's inner healer. Certainly the telepathic link at the beginning had been noted as a major point and the beginning of healing. It is quite feasible that additional information relative to breaking the trauma siege is telepathically passed to the patient at the same time as the information necessary to reactivate a senescence program or any other blockages in the innate healing intelligence.

Chapter 10

SENT HOME TO DIE

This case history touches something special in a different manner because it is a rare case involving two different forms of healing, including energy and information. Marie's was a tranquil life of house wife, mother and grandmother. Her needs were few and her pleasure was in caring for her expanding family. She lived within a strongly catholic country and community. She told me how she believed in God, Christ, the Immaculate Conception and she believed in spiritual healing and divine intervention and she was convinced I had been sent by God. Well, if explaining to the Spanish doctor what I understood my support healing posed some problems, then explaining neuroscience and telepathic conversations and innate healing systems intelligence with this dear woman, would not do either of us any favours.

When she was found to have cancer she was sent to hospital to have an operation to remove a small tumour from her stomach. During the operation the surgeons found the cancer had spread much further than they thought. The operation was terminated as the surgeon considered anything they could do would be too little too late. Afterwards, despite all efforts her operation wound would not heal but kept erupting in a yellow mess. Finally the doctors considered there was nothing else they could do that a nurse could not do on a home visit.

I was told that Marie was effectively sent home to die. The hospital couldn't justify her much needed bed any longer. A visiting nurse was organised to clean and dress her wound daily at her home. When I first saw Marie she was clearly weak. She was dressed and moved about the room slowly and clearly in some pain as she held her tummy as she walked. I explained the procedure I proposed based on intuitive guidance, then we went into Marie's bedroom, she lay on her bed. Five or six members of her family followed us and seated themselves around the room.

Marie had been through an awful experience and no doubt trauma shock of discovering her cancer. The operation and the aftermath had taken its toll. She had heard all the detail, the excuses or stories from the surgeons, doctors and nurses, so what could I tell her that would make any difference.

I knelt down in silence beside Marie, who seemed to be at complete peace and remarkably relaxed given a total stranger was about to do something of which she knew nothing about but I was forgetting her perfect faith in God.

This time, not only did I help Marie to enter into a very deep state of relaxation by hypnosis but I also entered a deep meditative like state while still holding Marie's hand. From that moment I had little recollection of what happened for the next three hours. When I had finished, I rested for more than an hour. Then I was taken to the kitchen to find Marie, quite a different person. She was full of energy, activity and freely moving around the kitchen, quite different than the person I had first met a few hours earlier. Alone she had prepared a feast to honour my presence that covered the large table in the middle of the room.

About a week later I received a telephone call saying within 24 hours Marie's wounds had healed completely. On various occasions further messages arrived confirming that Marie was in good health. Fifteen years later I received one last telephone call to say that Marie had died at the age of 75, of natural causes, following a full, active, happy and healthy life since my visit.

What can I say other than this was one of many cases, where little was said or exchanged other than whatever happened at the level of telepathy.

Chapter 11

WHEN A DOCTOR CAME CALLING

Naturally I must advise all to seek professional advice and help from the orthodox medical services. Just occasionally I found the medical profession turning the tables and came knocking on my door.

On one notable occasion my patient John had been described as suffering a major mental breakdown. He was a junior partner of a firm of solicitors. His wife Katherine was an extremely bright doctor and active professional in the medical training world. She had heard of my healing work and arranged an appointment in the hope of helping her husband. Various psychologists had done their best but little changed for John.

It was not unusual for a patient to be accompanied by their wife, husband, partner or a friend. The only problem in this case, was that when I asked John questions his wife would answer for him before he had a chance to speak for himself. John could hardly get a word in edgeways. In fact it appeared that in his wife's company he ceded all responsibility for himself as though a child again.

A mental breakdown is not something I would normally consider healing best suited to. As a rule I do not recommend any alternative healer delve into the field of diagnosis. In this case I was being consulted by a doctor, which was a little tricky as my trusted intuition indicated her husband was not really suffering with a mental breakdown. I felt there was no harm in running a deep relaxation process via hypnosis followed by coaching to see what came out of the process. When it came to the relaxation there was a continual flow of information from Katherine as to exactly what the problems were and what I needed to do.

Certainly John needed help but evidently whatever form that came in, if it was going to work then Katherine had to be included as she seemed to be part of the problem. As can be seen in theatrical staged hypnotic acts, an audience may witness a person being hypnotised without they themselves falling into an hypnotic trance. This demonstrates hypnosis is normally relative to a particular person on whom the hypnotist is focused. Such being the case the hypnotic focus was also focused on John's spouse. Within a few moments Katherine was resting quietly in an easy chair with her eyes closed. Her rapid eye movements; clearly seen beneath her eyelids; indicated even in an hypnotic state she was still trying to interfere. Nevertheless, peace and the session prevailed without further interruption. When later asked to open their eyes, instantly she realised what had happened. What had happened had clearly annoyed but intrigued her.

"*How did you do that?*" She demanded.

She immediately launched into a discussion about telepathy, hypnosis and healing, completely ignoring her husband and the reason for our meeting. Katherine's behaviour spoke volumes to me about her husband's condition. This was not judgemental of Katherine but raised the question of how compatible this couple really were. Now I was getting close to interfering, as such it was clear to me that healing was not right in this case but I did have life coaching as a healing fallback.

Later in a session without his wife, John explained how he had lost faith in himself and his reason to be. He fully accepted that no faith in himself meant no self confidence, which meant he had no driving purpose in life. Eventually no confidence in himself meant almost total incapacity to achieve the simplest of tasks no matter how much he wanted to. He seemed unable to do anything other than read the newspapers and watch television. He realised he was practically dysfunctional. The moment he mentioned the words, "wanting to but unable," and "no self confidence," when he had been a junior partner in London law firm, I recognised the typical symptoms of burnout. Free of his wife's interruptions and her personal interpretations, I began to recognise more of the classic symptoms of stress burnout. My conclusion was that John had become dysfunctional due to prolonged high stress mal-perceived by psychologists as a full blown mental breakdown. The stress had been going on for many years almost since the beginning of his marriage. He explained the stress had increased as his children grew up.

His stress was not only because of his wife domineering effect on his life but also because his two young children were so bright. Even they could out think and outperform him in almost everything in the home. In short his stress became supercharged as he believed he no longer had a purpose or role to play in the family. John explained how he had abandoned all personal goals, objectives or hope; also he had tendencies to suicidal thoughts but did not trust himself to go through with it.

This second meeting was a case of coaching pure and simple. I explained to John how I felt that healing in my normal format was not going to solve his problem but like healing, the coaching would guide him to finding his own best solutions. John agreed and we both accepted achieving this goal would, at its best, be a carefully planned long term strategy. As the coaching progressed, I saw a change in his thinking and renewed faith in himself as if he then understood a new way forward.

Previously being treated as a case of mental breakdown, John said he saw no future even though he could not explain why. However, accepting himself being in a state of stress burnout felt right to him also this somehow gave him hope. He said he felt I was the first person to understand what had really happened to him. John produced what he felt was a workable program, which would lead to getting himself into action again.

My question was simply, could he do it? This may have been an intuitive warning that John was going to stop the coaching too early. I am always worried when I lose contact with patients abruptly. Invariable they believe they are fixed but as in the case of Jim the businessman and the Spanish doctor, they may have no awareness of the challenges of the possible emotional aftermath.

John did regard himself better so he did stop the coaching and I did not hear from him for some months. Later he called me to explain he had stopped the coaching due to his parents who were psychologists not liking the idea of healing or life coaching. Although they had persuaded him to stop the healing/coaching, strangely this intervention proved to be a wakeup call that he was old enough to decide what was best for himself. John stopped the coaching as his parents wished but he had found sufficient support from the coaching to continue his plans without a word to anyone.

This change in strategy signified to me that he had rediscovered his faith in himself and awoken a defiant willpower in understanding what he wanted and to succeed in getting it. This signalled that John was on his way up. I had my concerns about him sliding back without any support. It was necessary not to interfere but rather allow him to take back control for himself. I made sure he was aware of the dangers to watch out for and asked for his assurance that he was willing to call me if he felt he was getting into any sort of trouble with his renewed progress.

There is no positive indicator of what is possible or inevitable. Only by having an open flexible mind to experiment, and test new ideas or concepts, can help any of us develop experience, confidence and trust in busting any personal impossibility myths.

Given the poor state John was in, I was impressed how in just three coaching sessions he had broken out of his own virtual prison sentence so quickly. From all indications, his parent's interference seemed to be the straw that broke the camel's back, which woke up his inner tiger with a jolt and with surprisingly fiery indignation. With the belief he was not a mental wreck but in some sort of semi-overwhelm approaching stress burnout state, this changed his life. This plus some coaching released his innate vision of the future. Suddenly he had his tiger by the tail so there was no stopping him even if that had been for his own good. Sometimes when healing proved to be spectacular like this it seemed too easy even if to the outside world it looks like doing the impossible. As this book progresses I explain how and why it really is easy, once the difficult part of learning has been achieved. This was establishing a strategy for how to do the right thing of never, never interfering and allowing a far greater innate healing intelligence do the hard or complicated work.

Experience and practice has taught me to recognise when a client has more work to do on their emotions, beliefs and attitudes before a healing will fully take place. I am always open to the possibility of a miracle as that inner shift or change could happen in just one word and one second of time. That one crucial word has the power and capability to touch an emotional blockage in the perfect way so that it is instantly released.

The perfect word has to be aligned with many other issues for the inner miracle of spontaneous healing to be triggered. This is not something to fear that it only happens by chance. One simple word will do, if it is the right one from the right person at the right moment.

One word in the right company of words can have the power to open the mind to enlightenment. That word can be so fundamental that in the course of a few seconds the mind reprocesses old redundant self-limiting beliefs and deletes them at the same moment replacing them with a greater or better truth. That flash of intuitive truth better supports a sense of reality and as in John's case, a renewed faith in himself blossomed once again.

This is an interesting case that demonstrates that John became his own healer the moment the words "mental breakdown" were exchanged for "burnout." I was not solely responsible for triggering John's inner tiger of recovery. His parents interfering once again in his life played their part in John's breakout.

That one change plus a few perfect words during the coaching aligned a new thinking process. They were the product of the telepathic communication rapport between me the support healer and the patient's subconscious intelligence. I mentioned at the beginning that on meeting John, intuitively I knew it was not a case of mental breakdown. This is an example of not interfering but being directed by the patient's innate healing intelligence. This is achieved by the patient's innate healing intelligence being the only intelligence to know exactly what is wrong and what was needed to kick start the inner healing process.

An example of the right word or words was when a mature woman of some considerable social standing was convinced she was dying of some invisible illness that even the best doctors in London could not identify. Intuitively or telepathically, I could not detect there was anything wrong with her. She was insulted by my assertions and became quite indignant. Intuitively the words, "you are as fit as a bull elephant" came into my mind. There was no way I was prepared to say such a thing to this special person, people have lost their heads for less. Nonetheless my intuitive guidance insisted. In a moment out it came. My patient's head spun around so fast I was worried she might have done herself an injury. *"Are you sure,"* she said. I confirmed my intuitive assertion. *"In that case that is perfect. Thank you for your forthright opinion."* Each Christmas thereafter for many years, I received a card confirming I had been right and that she continued to be in good health.

It is always striking when something like this happens. Another example that needed a little more time was that of Jim the entrepreneur briefly mentioned at the beginning of this book. The first day and half of coaching was clearly just preparing the ground. When the moment was right that perfect word appeared and like a missile it targeted his emotional blockage. Jim froze a second or two and then in one inspirational flash, everything he had been unable to see or understand before was immediately clear to him.

Dr. Deepak Chopra says;

"The body must be credited with an immense fund of know-how."

Chapter 12

THE KEY

W hat you will read and I hope find of interest in the following chapters on how the body is capable of healing itself, is an awareness of the balance and nuances of being available, understanding, intervening but not interfering. Despite a complex whole body/mind system; everyone has an amazing capability to manage that complexity without really knowing it exists, where it is or how it works. The principle inconsistency of support healing therapies of all descriptions is like everything in life, they all have their limits. The greatest challenge is that we never can know the limits of any therapy. Next is the difficulty that every human being is unique and therefore will respond to healing therapy in a uniquely different way. Thus, the important point is to understand that the innate healing systems and their associated centres of intelligence do actually exist, so best to learn how to support and work with and not against them.

In the beginning all we need to do is learn and practice a few basic rules. In a few words these rules can be wrapped up as follows. Stop getting in the way of this immense power and intelligence with the not so good things we mindlessly do without thought for our best mental, emotional and physical health. Cease activity in all those stressful things we do with our minds, largely by not being mindful of exactly how the mind works. Debunk redundant thinking practices and learn how to use the far greater power of our brains and subconscious minds to far better effect. Stop doing what we think is right before checking first. Finally ensure there is harmony and balance. Already I have indicated why a well managed mind is so relevant and critical to a healthy body. So often to achieve this we must recognise the important significance of inquisitive focus on so much we take for granted.

Consequently I resorted to being my own devil's advocate. This was to challenge myself to explain so much that over the years of healing research and development, I had taken for granted and as read. When one becomes closely familiar with a complex subject, especially where a great deal of intuitive and telepathic information is involved, it is too easy to assume others fully understand. Worse still is to limit explanation because one assumes others do not or will not understand.

During this process, I further understood to achieve my best during my life, I have no choice but to take back a little more of the responsibility for understanding the meaning of life and what makes me tick. Taking back the power of making the right choices for the right reasons is crucial to our greater success. Knowing ourselves and what really helps rather than hindering our own progress and sometimes that of associated others is fundamentally important. The main hurdle is we may take more notice of what is wrong with others, than we take notice of what could be improved in ourselves.

During support healing or any healing; within a very short time space; an enormous amount of information can be transferred telepathically from the healer to the patient and back again. If the therapist or support healer is giving advice he or she has not the remotest idea of how the patient's conscious and subconscious thinking works or the meaning taken from the healer's albeit well intentioned information. For this reason anything the healer believes to be true and helpful is pure and simple interference unless it is directly taken from the patient's or client's subconscious centres of intelligence and knowhow. This is the only way I have deduced it is possible to support, intervene and not interfere.

The main point in communicating with what is often referred to as a "higher intelligence," is to stop overloading the conscious mind. The secret is to work with the greater potential of the subconscious all knowing intelligence and thus without the usual stress. If we do not bother looking or do not use the flashes of intuitive inspiration that occasionally break out of the subconscious, it really is a case of, "if you do not use it, you lose it." One of the keys to manage the activating of spontaneous healing is in learning how to access and use this subconscious mind power on demand to its very best advantage.

Success depends on the vital procedures necessary for communicating the right information to the right place in the right way. During my support healing experiences; as complicated and impossible as it seems on the surface, learning about how the mind and body works was not an attempt to interfere but in knowing what I might do in order to be certain that I did nothing by error, accident or in any way assuming I knew what I was doing.

Unravelling this conundrum, I came to understand there was only one solution. This was I had to find the very best intelligence that understood precisely what was needed to effect a healing. The case studies within the text and the above and following chapters show how I achieved this also how powerful the inner healer is when it is supported and freed to work properly. Some of those case studies also show what can go wrong especially if the patient does not want to be healed. This may be a case of asking for healing while also having a secret agenda to not let it happen. In one case within the text, a woman was healed and then deliberately reversed the healing because she found the benefits to her life were greater as a permanent invalid. As you will read later she claimed she reversed it but I am not sure. As far as she was concerned, if her church friends believed she was still in pain that was all that was needed. Thus the support healer needs to be aware of consequences in the form of side issues. These may arise after the healing is successful in dramatic ways such as in the case of the Spanish Doctor.

Mark's case of crashing his racing car revealed patently clear insights into to how the healing was working because the results were apparent within minutes. In the beginning I admit to being taken aback because Mark was in a far worse state than I had been given to believe. On reflection I realised this degree of severity made no difference. This was simply because my job was to release his innate healing system that had become stuck. After it was free to work fully again, Mark completed his own healing himself.

Throughout the years of studying and analysing my support healing and past case histories, I came to understand that I had inadvertently developed a subconscious automatic support healing practice that was self activating. This momentarily stopped my conscious concerns so that I could access the all important intuitive and telepathic guidance. This meant I did not have to go through a process of consciously aligning myself perfectly with my patient or deciding how to act without interfering. Thus intuitively I immediately recognised and understood all that I had to do without the possibility of interfering.

This self activating subconscious automatic support healing became the basis for MindPower Recognition and Neuro-fault Protection automatic mind strategies for high performance. The first of these was a self activating safe driving strategy. The basic principle is this and other high performance subconscious programs work via self activating intuitive and telepathic intelligence. Once I realised there is no stress in the subconscious mind, this became the for-runner for all subconscious high performance thinking free of stress. This is explained in more detail in my book High Performance after Burnout.

In Mark's case, before I arrived, he had already healed the emotional blockages by accepting to let go of something very dear to him but could so easily have killed him. It was possibly the accident trauma level of severity that blocked his innate healing system intelligence from completing his own healing. It could be said that his innate healing intelligence had its own "want to but cannot syndrome." If you remember, standing in front of Mark, I telepathically asked his innate healing intelligence what it wanted me to do. Left to my own devices, I am certain I would have neither thought of the action I came to execute nor would I have dared to do something so challenging. This all points to the principle of the healer not interfering but being fully attentive to the patient's subconscious intelligence who is the only intelligence to understand precisely what is required of the support healer.

Within these case histories you will read about, how I began to have clues in answering my question why I had been called to those people, or they came to see me after everything in the orthodox medical chest had failed. First of all I had apparently inherited the necessary skills albeit there was room for a lot of learning and improvement. Second, I seemed to have a natural aptitude to adapt to just about any situation. Third, I was not restricted by bizarre beliefs of spiritual correctness. Forth, I had the freedom of an entrepreneur to be available also travel the country and abroad in the case where patients could not travel.

There proved to be a definite reason in the beginning for not needing to understand and then later needing to understand without trying to help or interfere. This was; as far as I can ascertain; a case of my own innate healing systems intelligence guiding me in a stage by stage learning of how I could achieve this subtle mix of being available, doing what was needed of me but not interfering. Therefore, only by careful analysis of each healing case, was I to eventually conclude that only by telepathic communications with the patient's subconscious inner healing intelligence could I play my full part in any healing event. The real healer, the patient's innate healing intelligence is 100% cognisant of precisely what is needed. It does not need any other outside intelligence. Hence, any helpful well meaning thoughts of my own were getting into that stream of information raises the possibility of inadvertently interfering and blocking the real healer.

I found it was not a case of saying sorry that was wrong, let's start again. Once the damage of breaking trust is done that is it, game over. The patient's innate healing intelligence simply shuts the entry door. This is exactly as we do when we lose trust in a service provider or a friend. We do not let them into our lives any longer. Furthermore it is likely that innate intelligence remembers. There are people who feel duty bound to help where help is not needed and this is perhaps the hardest thing to learn especially when activating spontaneous healing. This is the first principle of life coaching and NLP therapy. "Do not interfere and do not try to help," which are importantly equal to "do no harm."

The potential for one mistake, is the potential for one mistake too many. Thus the reason why so many support healers underperform is certainly because their patient's innate intelligence is wary of just one mistake. Usually the first mistake is already made in the healers mind in believing they are the healer.

A blockage within an innate healing system or thinking strategies can be any number of things. Limiting emotions such as doubt sends out signals the support healer is in a state of confusion about who they are and what they should be doing as a support healer. This also sheds light on the reasons why established reliable orthodox medical treatments may work for one patient but not all cases. This can be that the doctor has his or her doubts about the ultimate success of the treatment. Those thoughts are telepathically transferred to the patient, whose innate healing systems consequently shut out any possibility of the proposed treatment or even the innate healing system affecting a cure.

Having trained and continued studying sports mind coaching for high performance, I found the same principles apply as with support healing. This exact same principle is apparent in top sports performers and notably apparent in the case of golf players simply because of the nature of golf involving one person only. Therefore in such cases immediate results can be achieved just as the case of Mark, but without having to put them through a secondary pain trauma. I maintain that just as in support healing, in high performance golf coaching, unless the golfer fully allows their subconscious player to play the game, the golfer is playing against themselves and the course. If the golf player in fully in their subconscious intelligence they are playing with themselves and the course is helping them. This is; if they allow their subconscious golf playing intelligence to play the ball unfettered by conscious thoughts of how to play golf, the result can be extraordinary. However, the error of forgetting or failing to get into what is called the zone the result is as bad as it gets. Any conscious interference of the golfer thinking they know what to do, sets up a subconscious "want to but cannot syndrome." Then the ball continually ends up in the long grass and their name never gets to or it slips off the leader board.

To some the above may seem irrelevant until noticing that what is known as the Zone for sports people, also applies in high performance life coaching and support healing. They are all fundamentally the same process of working with the brain the way the brain likes to work or is capable of working at its very best.

In general telepathy is poorly understood and there is no broad based recognised training for developing telepathic skills for a wide range of purposes. Nonetheless, I have found that life coaching and NLP skills and training are useful in developing telepathic skills and thus creating the vital telepathic link with the client or patient. As I have already demonstrated it is particularly important for the support healer to understand the importance of telepathy in the healing process also how it prevents the support healer from interfering yet continuing to participating in the most appropriate way.

Therefore, essentially it makes little difference if it is a life coach with support healing training or a support healer with life coaching or NLP training and experience. This point demonstrates that any form of orthodox or alternative healing can be improved with the addition of life coaching, NLP and support healing methods. This is principally because these elements reduce stress and build the telepathic communications in the way the brain, mind and body intelligence centres like and are best able to work.

Talking with doctors and reading or listening to surgeon's memoirs, it is clear that a considerable number have taught themselves to speak to the patient's internal intelligence telepathically during an operation or afterwards while the patient is still sedated. One surgeon explained this by repeating what he telepathically says to his patients.

"I am the mechanic; it is you the patient who is the healer. I can remove what had turned bad and join the pieces together in the right way in order for your body to function more or less correctly. It is you who decides if it will be a success or a failure. My surgical team and I have done everything within our knowledge and power to fix your medical condition. Now the act of healing is in your hands to do your very best as your part of this team work."

Notice the surgeon is speaking to the patient telepathically. This is because he wants to speak to the patient's innate healing systems intelligence and not to the patient's conscious mind.

Andrew Weil M.D. says in the forward to his book 'Spontaneous Healing' *"A man whose lungs are filled with cancer is sent home to die, having been told that medicine can do nothing for him. Six months later he re-appears in his doctor's office, tumour free. A young woman diabetic, a heavy smoker – lies unconscious in a coronary care unit following a bad heart attack. Her doctor anguishes over the fact that her cardiac function is rapidly declining and he is powerless to save her. But the next morning she's awake and talking, clearly on the way to recovery. A neurosurgeon tells grieving parents that their son, who is in a coma following a motorcycle accident and severe head injuries, will never regain consciousness. The son is now fine."*

From all accounts as above, many doctors have one or maybe more stories of this sort of spontaneous healing against all the odds of survival. These demonstrate the power of the body's "Innate Healing Intelligence" when the doctors stand back and stop interfering knowing there is no more they can do. When interfering stops is when whatever was blocking healing; therefore blocking medical treatment; is reversed.

Recognising a patient's innate healing system intelligence can block or give the green light for healing is understandably troubling. Without understanding, respecting and catering for the emotional element, it all must seem totally irrational. The technology supporting the medical professionals is formidable and we look to them when we are in trouble. Not everyone surgeon or doctor is prepared to tell all for fear of being seen to act unprofessionally. They would not want to let the team down or burst the myth; thus destroying the trust we have come to have in them and in medical science.

Due to my contact with many nurses, indeed also a number of doctors during my NLP training, it became apparent that some hospital's senior nursing staff provide training to teach telepathically talking supportively to their patients as they carry out their caring and medical support skills. Until my NLP training I had not realised that some doctor's nurses and surgeon's were actively practicing this telepathic conversation as a purposeful means of bypassing the patient's own conscious thoughts of negative limiting beliefs. This is great because, "it does no harm" also it is precisely what I do as a support healer. Allied to this telepathic connection, surgeons, doctors and operating room nursing support staff understand that any comment of their worst fears for the patient's recovery can have a significant negative effect on the patient's recovery. Thus such talk may become an interference and risk of blocking the real healer from finishing the job successfully.

Dr Andrew Weil indicates, when the doctors have done their best and then let go, then innate spontaneous healing may take over to do the real healing. In which case, success against all the odds goes down to the overall skills and medical treatment. The subtle telepathic support and the patient's innate healing participation will inevitably remain unnoticed.

Paradoxically, miraculous spontaneous healing may occur because of an internal emotional shock on learning the hard negative truth or perhaps a hard but better truth. This seems to have occurred in the case history, "When a doctor came calling." The patient had been seriously undermined by being told he had suffered a mental breakdown. For him this meant the end of his life and essentially he was mentally damaged and broken and that was exactly how he began behaving. When he considered the possibility of overwhelming stress or burnout, he began making new understanding connections. As these were more compatible with his experience and his real state of mind, he was able to break the trauma grip of misinformation he had been in. Then spontaneously he began to take back responsibility for himself and move forward with his life.

The inner harmony and synchronisation needed to trigger spontaneous healing could be triggered by an anti-trauma trauma. This positive effect trauma is in that brutal statement saying there are no more medical options. That shock of hearing the truth; for possibly the first time; could be the emotional turning point that breaks down a limiting belief within the patient. Perhaps instead of falling into deeper conscious despair, the patient or their innate healing intelligence silently says to themselves something like;

"Oh really, well we will see about that, just stand back and watch this space."

We know that in the right circumstances, what may appear as a hard unremitting inevitability to some can be provocation into action to others. This brutal truth jolt, this wake-up call to the system can be the greatest of all motivators to our conscious thoughts and actions. Doing that with the conscious mind, this quantum shift is possibly the vital key to alerting and goading our greater innate healing intelligence into action.

Look carefully at the above and compare it with all I have said about support healing. Supporting the non interference rule exists in successful medical practices. As the surgeon said, "he is the mechanic." He is doing what the body and its innate healing system apparently cannot do. When we analyse what surgeons do and what post-surgery healing means and entails, it becomes clear that surgeons do not heal, the best they can do is make it possible for healing to take place by removing what is physically blocking the patient's natural body healing processes.

A surgeon cannot put back the spark of life and the capability for the body to heal itself if that spark is hell bent on extinguishing itself. Given this inevitability, surgeons and doctors have little power to guarantee healing without the full support of the patient's subconscious will to live, keep their immune system in good shape and capable and their innate healing intelligence free to do its job.

Therefore, to the best of my understanding and experience, support healing first of all underpins the body's innate healing intelligence to clear any of its own blockages. That is so it can do what it says on its label. That does not mean there is ever a time to interfere with what any support healer thinks is right or what is a perfect remedy. We can never do this successfully because there is no means of understanding the incredible complexities involved within the innate healing system. Because every living human being is unique, having their very personal DNA programs, beliefs and values, any well meaning ideas or intentions of healing are inevitably interfering. Those healers of whatever genre, including life coaching and NLP therapy are at great risk of over participating by irresponsible intervening and thus interfering.

The reason why as a support healer, I found myself so often to be the last resort is because our trust and first port of call is always with the official medical system. As I have demonstrated, support healing can play a formidable role. An example is the case of the young boy undergoing dialysis but for unknown reasons something was blocking his treatment so he was slipping into a coma. The doctors were powerless. This case is much like that of Mark and The Rock. I did not try to communicate with their conscious minds but went straight to seek the guidance of their subconscious intelligence. Shortly after I had the intuitive feeling my job was done and I left the hospital. Immediately the boy began to respond to his treatment.

Participating and intervening must be associated with doing what is essential such as a surgeon or doctor repairing anything the innate healing system cannot repair itself. In the case of a support healer's participation, the only acceptable intervention is the telepathic communication and intent of being available to the specific guidance of the patient's innate healing intelligence, no more, no less.

Some people may argue there are circumstances where the line between intervening and interfering can be extremely fine therefore it is inevitably going to be crossed. This may be the case for the medical profession but certainly not in the case of support healing. Proving this without the slightest doubt may be difficult. The reason is the innate healing systems intelligence appears to understand exactly what it needs emotionally in the form of outside support to sustain its own spark of life and healing. Therefore, it is extremely sensitive to any error, deviation and thus interference. In surgery for all sorts of reasons unintentional minor errors can occur but because they are mechanical they can be corrected.

Like the research into senescence programs, the above information is based on experience, observations and an emerging logic, which occurs in probably all methods of medical research. It is all down to experience and circumstantial evidence involving the repetition of the same cycles of events followed by a positive healing. In other words, recognising what works, understanding how it can work and successfully repeating that learning.

It is not just the innate healing intelligence that understands precisely what the appropriate healing should be. Looking at the case of Mark the racing car driver, no surgeon worth his salt was prepared to operate on him. They all understood that operating to relieve his infirmity and pain would be inappropriate interference. I am certain the surgeons knew because nothing was broken nothing needed repairing. I am certain they all understood the pain was caused by his spinal column being distorted and squeezing the spinal cord due to and held in place by traumatised muscles. Therefore, they understood the solution was in getting all the muscles that had locked up to unlock by their own means. That; as my osteopath told me has to come from the inside and can be exceedingly difficult by technical methods. Therefore the question is what is controlling the muscles that can so ably resist external efforts to solve the problem. This blocking device can only be emotional trauma. An example of which was demonstrated by the junior solicitor's trauma of being convinced and believing he had had a mental breakdown and therefore he was broken. The moment he was given an escape route to believe otherwise, he healed himself. The speed of his breakout and renewed personal drive was remarkable.

I am not sure those specialists and doctors had been completely candid with Mark or he deliberately chose not to listen, understand or remember. Very possibly their advice, "of time will probably be his best healer," was very likely exactly what Mark did not want to hear. So long as he could get into the driving seat of a racing car, he could avoid the fact staring him in the face that he was getting too slow in his reactions and too old to drive racing cars. I also believe he was addicted to the adrenalin rush when driving. This was just as I had deduced my own addiction to adrenalin had occurred in my personal case of build-up to burnout. I did not have a racing car to hit a bridge to stop me, all I had, was the wisdom, intelligence and power of my innate survival and self protection intelligence. This suggests subconscious intelligence determines the ideal stopping strategy relative to the cause and thus indicating the appropriate method of healing.

The physical and emotional trauma to Mark's spine induced not just terrible pain but what I believe to be the Survival and Self Protection intelligence activating its "Do not ever do that to yourself again syndrome," and thus "The want to but cannot syndrome." It had just reason for this behaviour because Mark had been ignoring intuitive warnings to stop racing for some time. So why did Mark need to hit a bridge? My conclusion is that if he had simply hit burnout he would have forced his way through, driven again and possibly killed himself.

I personally experienced a similar event of traumatised muscles when skiing on packed and frozen snow. Saving those not familiar with a long explanation of what catching a wrong ski edge means, essentially, I tripped over my own skis while travelling at about 40mph, on a patch of ice when obliged to stop quickly on a tight turn. Actually, I did not just trip and fall over; due to my speed and sudden halt, my body was forcibly slammed onto the hard icy surface. By the evening my back and shoulders were seriously painful. Nothing short of high intensity electric shock treatment at a local clinic would undo my traumatised shoulder muscles. In this fall there was no emotional trauma that needed to be resolved other than perhaps a quickly forgotten embarrassment as my ego was seen to have made an embarrassing mistake in front of an entire advanced fast downhill ski class and my instructor. Ouch! But yes, the same innate message is, "do not do that again." Perhaps like Mark, my reactions were getting too slow indicating I was getting too old for the rigors of advanced fast downhill skiing. For Mark it was a bridge, for me it was a thick sheet of ice? Once emotional syndromes are set in motion, the innate healing intelligence seems to automatically determine whether the underlying problem is being addresses or not. The answer to this determines whether the innate healing systems will work with or against any form of treatment. Fortunately for me it did.   It could be argued that mark's accident was his own special form of burnout because his innate survival intelligence knew he would not willingly stop racing cars. Likewise, my own burnout was possibly because my innate survival intelligence knew I could not willing stop running my businesses and destroying my own life.

This case further cements my view as to how this level of support healing can play an important part in a team work situation. That is, in making a link between the surgeon or doctor and the patient's subconscious and innate healing intelligence. This is particularly poignant if we consider that cancers also fall into this same category. This is demonstrated in the cases of "The Spanish doctor and Sent Home to Die." After surgeons, doctors and nurses had done their best, the cancers remained uncontrollable. Only when the perfect support had removed the one most important limiting emotional factor, did healing of the cancers take place.

I am not qualified to comment on how the surgeons or doctors had intervened in these cases. All I can say is that my participation of support healing turned all that around exceedingly quickly. In both cases the patient's were able to re-invigorate their original spark of life and their innate healing intelligence.

Reading The Healer Within by Dr. Stephen Locke M.D. was when I first learnt about the body's innate healing intelligence and recognised its importance and connection to the healing I was doing. Quickly it made sense to not interfere but intuitively work with the patient as I had been doing. At least I understood why the spiritual healing methods were more smoke and mirrors than real healing.

Before my introduction to this innate healing intelligence, I had been given to understand the patient was supposed to have faith in the healer, and spiritual intervention whatever form that came in. Now I understood if healing was going to happen, I had to have absolute confidence in the patient's inner healing intelligence having faith and confidence in me not interfering.

Innate centres of intelligence like intuition, emotional intelligence, telepathy, explicit creative intelligence and others are important in what might be called preventive healing. When it comes to our health, to give ourselves to myth, superstition and magic, we step into a world of confusion, error, limitation and even subliminal fear. Our, minds and health are too important to make mistakes with. Thus, it is crucial to search for, if not the whole truth at least a greater truth than current levels of common hearsay or happenchance provide. This is all about who and what we really are, also what motivates us to undertake both good and not so good acts or performance.

When many of my patients came for healing, I am aware some did not respond as hoped such as I have indicated in the case histories above. Many patients; for whatever reason; I never saw or heard from them again. I can only presume by the law of averages that some did not heal. Some did forward feedback of the outcome by letters and postcards from near and far off places. If feedback did not come directly then a number of previous patients sent friends and acquaintances they felt confident to refer to me for healing. Such as the case of Mark, and Marie in Sent Home to Die, I would receive positive feedback by telephone or often a Christmas card indicating continued success of those earlier healings.

There are those healings that were distinctly different. Like Mark the Racing Car Driver, The Spanish Doctor and Telepathy with a Rock, these amounted to quantum leaps in learning something important about brain, telepathy, mind power and the inner healing intelligence. From these cases, I became aware of an amazing tenacity to live when by all accounts they should have slipped away days or even weeks earlier. I am thinking of the Rock in Telepathy with a Rock and my second visit to the Spanish doctor also the case of José in Christmas at Home. Those cases stick in the mind because they reveal an enormous amount of insight and provoke a great deal of thought and desire to better understand all that the brain and mind can do when there is something so important to pass on or something to finish. Such cases are extraordinary sometimes because of their special quality of simplicity and other times because of their emotional complexity.

Amusing things happened that led to learning about myself also about self-leadership. My reputation had preceded me yet the look of hopelessness was clearly visible on Mark's face. His condition was far more serious than I had been told. It was clear to me he did not expect anything out of the farce about to be enacted. Momentarily I sensed that prehistoric need to run for my life. Having Scotty beam me up to the Star Ship Enterprise would have been very nice. As this was unlikely to happen, disappearing through a crack between the highly polished floorboards beneath my feet would have been a good second option. Then I forgot my fears as everything slid into place spontaneously.

In minutes one of the most amazing healings I have been involved with was over. Mark's case was so significant because it was literally a case of *"pick up thy bed and walk."* Christina and Quarry Workers certainly was remarkable as it happened quickly and in front of all the neighbours. Mark's case, although no house full of neighbours, was so striking as there was no doubt before I arrived he could not walk and any movement resulted in terrible pain.

Christina's stress was invisible yet everyone knew it was very real. When she popped her cork of stress everyone heard and immediately understood the reasons why she had suffered so much and for so long. For me the reasons why the support healing had worked were quite clear. As for Christina's family and neighbours, I have no idea what they thought. These were people of simple needs and a strong faith in God, Jesus and miracles and now they had their very own experience to bolster their beliefs and to talk about as they sipped their wine in shaded kitchens away from the burning sun.

Writing it here it seems so easy. In fact it was easy and that is an important key to doing anything in life that is absolutely right. At the same time it was far from easy because there was a lot of learning and precisely training myself in how to do that. Of course another important key is being the right person at the right time doing the right thing, most importantly doing that free of any error at all.

I am conscious of the limitations involved in someone attempting to do the same thing without adequate training. The biggest obstacle is in first wanting to be the healer. This quickly invites the error of wishful thinking. It is so easy to mentally construct as imaginary guidance what is in fact no more than interference by inappropriate wishful well meaning. One of the most important aspects of true intuitive and telepathic intelligence on, which support healing depends, is being absolutely sure they are the real thing and not imposters to satisfy the ego.

So often I see people being lauded for their tremendous effort and courage but they are bemused as to what all the fuss was about. To them, they were just doing their job or what came naturally. To do this requires a depth of knowledge, considerable experience, absolute focus and open to trusting and knowing ourselves with an unshakeable confidence. We all can do this. Because we do not notice, because it was so easy, we did whatever was necessary quite automatically. In other words our conscious fears, doubts or other limiting beliefs or habits were not getting in the way, interfering or making a nuisance of themselves. Despite the challenges, we did not notice because we had automatically slipped into our zone state of subconscious competence of high performance. It is times like these that prove there is no fear or other limiting emotions or stress within the subconscious mind.

The process of conscious learning, practicing, changing, developing, testing, changing, practicing, testing again and recycling around and around until we finally get it right, certainly works. Yet within this process we are at great risk of learning inbuilt errors. This is flying in the face of our greater capability. It is all for the want of understanding how the mind works. In today's fast moving world of instant everything, in following this outdated process and taking too long, we risk missing the bus of opportunity and that without any doubt results in more and completely unnecessary errors and stress.

I appreciate stepping into this other dimension of subconscious intelligence can cause some uncertainty and mistrust by old thinking performance standards. On occasions I am conscious of spontaneously and telepathically alerting a total stranger's innate healing intelligence that they had a problem that needed fixing. Without a word of contact some would look at me after as if they understood something for a fleeting moment and then it had gone. Only by the deed of wanting to understand how my support healing worked could such a thing as I call support healing on the hoof possibly manifest itself.

I remember being on holiday somewhere in southern Portugal. I had joined a busy sidewalk alongside a crowded narrow old town street. An elderly woman was hobbling along in the street just a few feet ahead of me. We were in a dense crowd of people heading towards a summer spectacle in the town square. The old woman was bent double while supporting herself with a walking stick. In the past I have seen many elderly people suffering the same condition with their backs rounded with, curvature of the spine, largely due to a life of hard work, age, arthritis and stress. There should have been nothing exceptional about this woman other than I found myself speaking telepathically with her.

I was aware of my thoughts, *"Why are you walking like that when there is nothing wrong with you?"* This even surprised me, as all outward appearances were quite to the contrary.

What happened next was so spontaneous I was momentarily shocked. The old lady took two more steps, half straightened; hesitated a second between strides and then stood bolt upright. Her forward march stalled momentarily as she turned and looked directly into my eyes. Instantly she faced forward as the pressing crowd moved her onwards. As remarkable as it seems she just kept walking. The habit of relying on the walking stick prevailed. After two or three pointless attempts at bending to place the walking stick on the ground she walked on upright with the stick held by her side.

That event was no coincidence; I believe it is another demonstration of how simple healing can be when the right person at the right time spontaneously doing the right thing without interfering. This is what I mean by my healing experiences at times being so easy, but without experiencing it, who else would believe such a thing is even possible?

The above unsolicited spontaneous healing reminds me of a senescence program that being turned off, it cannot alert its cell intelligence to fix itself. If that is the case, my simple act of asking the elderly woman's subconscious intelligence the perfect question at the right moment, was all it took to make a major difference to her own innate healing intelligence.

Without interfering my telepathic question alerted her innate healing intelligence to something it was not aware of. This was likely because walking as if she had curvature of her spine had happened gradually over a number of years so it had become her normal limiting habit to walk in that bent fashion. This may have been due to the phenomena where we limit our performance either by fear, the fear of pain or possibly hereditary limiting expectations. In this case it could have been that this woman watched her own mother turn this way in old age. The pain may exist but no more than a twinge. It is often for the fear of pain that does not actually exist that we develop limiting habits to protect ourselves from the fear and put up with the inconvenience of what we believe we have to do. For this reason, I later concluded the woman was not crippled in the true sense of arthritic disfigurement. I kept an eye on her though she seemed fine. The summer show and music and fireworks exploded into life as we got to the town square, people pressed in ever closer and then apparently as my job was done, I lost her in the crowd.

Later when thinking about this incident, I remembered I had done the same thing for myself many years earlier while learning to walk on a narrow beam during a gymnastics class at my school. To start with, I repeatedly fell off the beam held only a few inches above the floor. For some reason I stood back and said to myself, "why do I need to fall off the beam?" When it was my turn to try again, intuitively I reminded myself, the objective of the exercise was to balance and not to fall. That internal question; the type of, which is now common in high performance life coaching, NLP therapy, also sports mind coaching; provided the precise information in the right place and right way that made all the difference. This changed my focus on balancing not the fear of falling and thus ensuring I would lose my balance. Without that self limiting fear, I was able to walk the length of the beam with ease. This illustrates the fact that when we allow fear to control, by mind freeze, we focus our attention on doing precisely what we do not want. If this should be a constant fear of a serious illness like cancer, heart attack or stroke, because that is what happened to a parent, this type of mind freeze gets us stuck in being the victim or invalid.

There is a similar self-defeating fact that the immune and innate healing systems can with the wrong input turn against the body with devastating effect. What is clear is the evidence that fears and limiting beliefs, however they are formed or from wherever they are gleaned, like unhelpful dogma, they can destroy all types of performance. This certainly applies to our own health performance. The support healing effect of life coaching, NLP and sports mind-coaching are particularly effective in correcting little understood limiting belief glitches in personal, professional.

What I have been demonstrating above is that our immune and self healing systems intelligence can also be vulnerable to performance glitches. Therefore I have no doubts that pre-emptive-healing like preventative homeopathic or acupuncture treatment is certainly a viable option for our general wellbeing and high performance.

Sian Beilock of the University of Chicago refers to the bad effects of doing so many wrong things to ourselves like stress when he says that: *"bad mistakes and brain freeze under pressure and stress is like a computer with too many programs running at the same time so it crashes."*

This process of crashing confidence can be seen in competition both in professional or amateur levels. This is where a sportsperson loses their zone or winning performance focus in favour of conscious doubt or fear and then in seconds their performance deserts them like rats leaving a sinking ship.

In the past fifteen years, neuroscience has opened a window into how brain functions really do work. In his book "Human Brain; How Smart Can You Get?" Sian Beilock talks about many new strategies being tested to calm nerves and mind freeze. These strategies are after treatment designed to concentrate on calming fast heart beat rate and reducing the production of cortisol also regaining better confidence with clearer thinking after the event.

The difference about Neuro-fault Protection strategies is to catch stress reactions like stressors and stress as early as possible before they become established and do their damage to performance. This is a preventive strategy not after treatment. In this process it is important to recognise how stress varies from a slow build up to an instant emotional reaction.

Stress may be piggybacking on an established bed of earlier compound stress. No conscious and wilful training or determination can spot an emotional reaction and stop it within less than one thousandth of a second. This is only possible with specialised subconscious mind programs, which work with pre-set automatic mechanisms in place designed to detect the coming dangers before they appear. These programs are created in the style of a radar system to spot and intercept stress and stressors long before they are capable of doing any harm.

Now there is the possibility of creating all manner of preventive health strategies; the same as designed for professional or sports purposes. These are designed to guard against a susceptibility to emotional traumas, stress and default mistakes thinking, whether or not they are associated to sports, careers, to cancers or other life threatening conditions. Preventive surgery of the type mentioned above for hereditary diseases has been reported as being a growing trend over the past several years. I realise modern medicine must be seen to come up with answers even drastic ones. The problem is that when the emotion of fear enters the equation, even when there is no proof greater than suspicions, one falls prey to emotional driven self mutilation. Earlier I mentioned if we are not careful how the mind plays games with itself. We are prone to fearing and sweating over what might have happened rather than accepting what did not happen. It is a short emotional step to falling prey to what might happen in the future even though there is no more evidence than presumptions.

Dr Deepak Chopra says the body has the intelligence to produce all pharmaceutical medications the pharmaceutical companies can. Maybe this is true, yet we all know that capability does not always function as it seems it should. So clearly our inner healing intelligence is some way from being all singing and all dancing for all occasions. Therefore the key to changing this imperfect state is to care more about who we are, how we work, what is best for us and what we can do to protect and help ourselves from unseen dangers.

One thing we must always keep in mind is that the brain/mind can work for or against our best intentions with equal force. For example, when in a state of anxiety or particularly high stress, those emotions act on the amygdala gland in the limbic system very fast indeed. The consequences are many and varied. Sian Beilock says,

"When the amygdala is over active with strong anxiety emotions, it can disrupt clear thinking."

Forewarned is certainly forearmed but what are the risks of jumping the gun. In 2015 a famous American actress grabbed world news headlines for a very unusual reason. She had both her healthy breasts removed for the fear she might die of breast cancer as happened to her mother. For most women this is a drastic course of action. Nonetheless, the wilful mutilation of a healthy body in this way shows the power of emotional fear. What I am concerned about is that even if she is totally secure in the belief she now has no risks of breast cancer, every day of her life she will be looking for any signs of cancer in any part of her body. That may be to such an extent it can become a self fulfilling prophecy due to the mind's capability to fulfil that, which we focus on. Although she has had the main area of risk removed, the story may not be over. The tragedy is that with the aid of surgeons she may have possibly set herself up to fail. It is certain she will be focusing on what she does not want. As the brain cannot distinguish negative focus from positive focus, her focus on not wanting any cancers to appear is tantamount to setting in motion sufficient and sustained, stress inviting that very thing to happen.

Chapter 13

RECONNECTING THE BODY'S INNATE HEALING SYSTEM

S uccess starts with self-respect and self-support. Everything we can do to support the immune and innate healing systems such as controlling stress and body inflammation, all count to a more comfortable and therefore a more successful life. All being well, the inner-healing process is something the mind and body does quite naturally. This is not by some mysterious magic; these systems are managed by an incredible set of intelligence programs; provided we do not interfere but allow and support them to do their job. You will see in the next chapters more about how this miracle works every second of your life from beginning to end.

There are many reasons why the body's own healing process becomes confused, blocked or stops working in specific areas. Some of those reasons are due to the environment, some emotional and others are behaviours hidden from view in our DNA and chromosomes because our body systems are controlled by information and new information. Any changes due to new information have consequences. One estimate suggests that although this slows down in later years due to aging, approximately four million cells in the body are dividing every second. This means their complex DNA blueprints and their management programs are being copied and replicated at the same rate.

In a nut shell research shows that with every cell division there is the potential for small imperfections to major errors to occur that may result in cells going rogue (benign tumours) and some eventually becoming malignant tumours. For the most part; although currently conjecture; all those errors are being corrected by the innate healing system before anything gets seriously out of hand. But this process has no defences against such issues as emotional, chemical or radiation traumas. This is the first reason why to know ourselves and to keep ourselves in good fettle makes a great deal of sense beyond the obvious of protecting ourselves from the more common issues. The key to this is possibly focusing on improving and sustaining good health for the sake of good health. If that focus changes to the greater fear of falling ill or poor health because that is what happened to ancestors, friends or others know to them that will likely be precisely what will happen.

It then becomes an emotional issue and that is the worst kind. Seeking help for emotional issues is no longer a question of being a weakling or wimp; it is a matter of maintaining a life balance particularly keeping stress under control. It is a matter of being wise and strong in caring for the fact we have responsibilities and vulnerabilities we do not understand. When we cover up our vulnerabilities is when we lose sight of knowing ourselves. When we allow this to happen is when we begin to make more excuses than achievements.

In a notorious and highly publicised South African trial during 2015 and 2016, a father heard the account of his beautiful daughter being cut down in her prime by her boyfriend's irresponsible behaviour. Having seen this man immediately after the incident I did not recognise him three years later. This man's face and body language was a stark reminder of the destructive power of negative emotions stress. What had been previously a strong man was three years later an emotional and physical wreck. For me this is an example of the man's spark of life itself coming under attack of unimaginable trauma. Having suffered the stress trauma of being reminded of his daughter's futile death on a daily basis throughout the trial, this stress was without a doubt responsible in bring about a stroke and one if not two heart attacks.

Sometimes we do not have the choice if the emotional traumas we have to face are so terrible they go beyond our comprehension or ability to manage. It was clear in watching and listening to this broken father, he no longer had the choice of how he could behave. The negative emotion was the tail wagging the dog from the inside out until he looked more like a head-on express train crash victim than his former robust self. It is widely understood that emotions, stress and especially traumatic emotional stress changes behaviours. Whatever support he had received, to me it was clear the emotional trauma had taken over control of his mind and body in such a marked and most terrible way; it was challenging for me to watch.

Certainly in our modern societies it is difficult to know what to believe as there is so much information available on the subject of what is or is not healthy for our bodies and minds. For those taking any notice, much of that often conflicting information overload, must be accepted as most likely coming from vested interests wanting to promote their beliefs, values, products or services. It is important to note in these cases some of the information may be exaggerated even distorted by dubious motives. When reading a new research article in a journal or magazine, always, we need to be aware to note who funded the research or the real motives for writing the article. These will give a clue as to where the biases, distortions or the lies might have originated. The difficulty for us is the fact there will always be grains of truth even wisdom, somewhere within the deliberate misinformation. This has never been so well illustrated than during the 2016 American presidential election run-up, which ended in giving American journalism a very bad name.

Years ago when genes were beginning to be understood, it was considered they were fixed within each generation and passed from father to son and mother to daughter or vice versa. Darwin told us that genes take many generations to undergo change. This concept is now known to be misleading in that parts of gene information are being changed constantly even though that may not be outwardly apparent. This means not only new gene patterns are being created and passed to our children within our own life time; we ourselves never stop changing our DNA information. The fact is we do have and can have a greater specific and chosen influence on those changes. The food we eat, the work we do, the environment we live and work in, the beliefs, values and behaviours we stand for and live by, the large or small traumas even those we hardly notice, are all things that mould who we are and what we achieve. Those changes are gradually and indelibly imprinted into our DNA. These are the changes that cause us to change our thinking, grow mellow, wise and not rise to temptation, risk taking or anger so easily as years before.

Until the industrial revolution, apart from the trials and tribulation of life, things changed very slowly for most people. There was little chance to cross social, professional or life style boundaries preset by family position and inheritance. Notably the development of the humble peddle bicycle, all that began to change. This one invention proved to be a social game changer. The invention of the bicycle permitted the more adventurous to change old habits. Many began travelling further afield under their own steam. This meant they met new people and experienced things they had not seen or heard of before. Once the steam train was invented and passenger travel became possible, entire families began travelling distances never before imagined. This led to many more people travelling to find new employment and start a new life. One of the effects was that previously isolated communities began mixing, socialising; externally marrying on a regular basis and that meant more people went to live in a different location. This resulted in a significant change in the spread of previously locked up gene pools. This caused people to think in a new ways and adapt to new behaviours and habits. These changes that to us in the twenty first century seen as absolutely normal, were in those days shocking, chaotic and stressful. However they were crucial elements in the dynamics, which underpinned and fundamentally drove new thinking. From those changes came new ideas that made the industrial revolution the success it was.

Today everything is changing so fast, if we cannot change all but the most fundamental values practically on a daily basis, we are at high risk of being left behind by our children, family, friends and in our careers. This is essentially what happened in the case of "A doctor came knocking." Changing is stressful but should be short term. Worst is that in not changing we are in danger of suffering ever higher stress over a longer time frame. In this case his children were so bright at six and eight years old they could out smart him in just about anything simply because he did not accept that he had to change to meet his children's' needs. His values that children should be seen and not heard and certainly not challenging him or being brighter than their father was for him simply unacceptable.

The result was he opted out of his responsibilities and that became a slippery slope of opting out of life itself. That left him in a state of limbo and confusion where he became; for all intents and purposes ineffectual. Thousands of people suffer the same fate of losing touch with themselves and their changing world. The less fortunate may be seen sleeping in cardboard boxes in the streets and under bridges. In their own form of burnout they descend into the cave of their Survival and Self protection so deeply they never find their way out again.

The outward, material changes are difficult enough. Though not new, the emerging dominant stressors "the-new-kids-on-the-block" are growing pollution, unseen hazardous chemicals, artificial hormones in foods and domestic products, industrial and commercial misinformation, global warming, growing corruption and now wide distrust in the political systems and to cap it all a growing rise in social disorder and terrorism. The solution to these problems is to understand this is the new order. Certainly for the elderly but for us all it is better to be current with these affairs than shutting them out completely. Shutting them out denies a truth and that creates its own distortions, which leads to disconnection, seclusion or a reclusive mentality and that may possibly lead to heath problems. Seclusion is bad enough for the human spirit. Disconnection from life sends a powerful message to all innate centres of intelligence that there is no will to be part of life, from there on it is a slippery downward slope.

Substances like artificial food flavour enhancers, colourings and packaging containing chemicals that mimic hormones like oestrogen and much more are stressful because they are to be found everywhere, thus they are difficult to avoid. Plastic pollution is now so catastrophic our seas are polluted with anything from micro fragment to complete plastic bags that are ingested into the fish we eat. Thus, in this naturally recycling world, we get our discarded rubbish delivered right to our dinner plates. We either cause ourselves stress by not doing our best to change or we live with the growing stress of what we did before because it is easier. The "catch 22" is if we fail to change. By avoiding the issue and the default option, we eventually get something more stressful as we learn to live with what we do not like or want.

Whether by choice or default, whatever the changes in our lives, they are causing a change in our genes by a drip – drip process over months and years. This is far faster than many centuries of family generations have done in the past. These are perhaps minor compared to the stresses of succeeding in our studies, qualifying, training and constantly retraining in our professions. Living with and managing a life based on insurmountable debt, maintaining social status and ever greater demands for higher performance has its hidden consequences. Getting and staying ahead of this vicious cycle has its own rewards but also its stresses.

Tim Spector says in his book 'Your Genes Unzipped' *"As for our human urges, addictions and cravings, admitting to yourself that you have innate genetic impulses, is the first crucial step to dealing with life's problems. Everyone has a different set of drives, strengths and weaknesses. Recognising the various forms they take is important so that you can focus on alternative and less damaging reward strategies that your body and brain need to keep themselves happy – without harming or killing ourselves too early."*

Tim Spector uses the words *"innate genetic impulses,"* these words mean genetic programs already imprinted in our DNA and passed down by our ancestors. In effect they are the puppet master of our habitual behaviours including thinking behaviours. Failing to change many of this means, we become responsible for wrong-footing ourselves with the result of far too much unnecessary stress.

The subject of DNA and genes is complex. It may be easier to think of these things as construction and maintenance manuals containing hundreds of thousands if not billions of operational programs or best practice guide lines and blue prints. These blue-prints manifest themselves especially in our numerous centres of intelligence such as innate healing, emotional and survival and self protection intelligence. They are the drivers of how we appear physically, our characters, our capabilities and skill preferences, subliminal beliefs and values. These are different from those we choose ourselves either deliberately or by default. They determine our health weaknesses, strengths and much more. Some of those programs have an influence on our internal healing process thus, the more we understand about the subject the more we get to "know ourselves." As Tim Spector says know our *drives, strengths and weaknesses* thus the more we can help ourselves and our better health.

In his book "Your Genes Unzipped" explains not only how many ailments or health conditions occur in this way but also alien ancestral attitudes or behaviours, and states of mind and thinking patterns all amounting to who we are. As stated at the beginning of this book, Greek philosophers said, "to know yourself first know your mind." Lest you forget, perhaps it is worth adding, "know our ancestor's minds beliefs and values and then begin making some comparisons with our own values a century or two later." Just knowing where our ancestors lived, what their professions were, any photographs, letters or other indicators such as heirlooms, medals, miniature paintings, birth, marriage and death certificates and a whole host of other information, all give many clues to their beliefs and values and thus how well they achieved knowing themselves also what they passed on to us that we do not know about.

By doing so, one may just begin to understand more about our mysterious behaviours, stumbling blocks in life or perhaps the good and not so favourable gifts we were born with. This is if we have not bothered to notice the signs pointing to them. When we become well aware of our not so favourable behaviours we might like to change them. We may have yearnings to try something like playing an instrument, singing, painting, acting, sailing, etc. This level of knowing our origins can alone change a life by virtue of realising how some capabilities that might have disappeared long ago still exist due to DNA coding passed down the line.

Life is not about waiting for things to fall in our laps, sometimes we have to go digging for what can make a difference by our own efforts. A tendency to have a bad temperament is exactly the same, yet this is not normally referred to as a gift. DNA coding is how those ancient habits are the invisible but durable strings that control unexpected performance both good and bad. DNA coding is just a challenging puppet master that automatically fires up outdated reactions to any of the multitude of stressors continually popping in and out of our lives.

Tim Spector's book "Your Genes Unzipped" combined with Anne Ancelin Schûzenberger's book "The Ancestor Syndrome," makes a powerful bridge between the science of our genes and the very real practicality of knowing our ancestors. This is done through guided telepathy and linking onto the field of energy and all information. The consequence can be the start of changing at least some of the less desirable personal traits we know about and possibly some we have not noticed or choose not to notice. This also shows how taking a peek into the lives and thinking processes of our ancestors; how they shaped or influenced the past and present; thus how they will make or mar our own future and achievements.

Anne Ancelin Schûzenberger says, *"We build up knowledge and memories through accumulation of unresolved conflicts, hatred, revenge, vendettas, of secrets of what is unspoken. At the unconscious level these and many other emotional memories are passed to our children via transgenerational transmission – hidden memories transported within family genes. The main objective is to look for repetitive behaviour traits or patterns, good and bad alike. Likes, dislikes - terrible events or traumas in the past may give you important information about how and why you think the way you do."*

If the family history is difficult to come by, one relatively simple exercise anyone can do at any time in their lives is to analyse their successes and failures. We may accept these but do we understand them? The reason why is so we become fully cognisant of what works and why and then when and where to repeat the best of them and do our best to control those that are not so perfect.

This issue is important; it is also a simple recipe to remember. A good balance of life brings with it better health and happiness. The proof of the pudding is that successes results in more feel-good hormones and more profitable ideas. Discord and failures produce more stress and cortisol than clear thinking.

Because each body and mind is conditioned by its own unique genetic code of transgenerational programs, each one of us has a unique health profile. This profile dictates the aches, pains, illnesses or health conditions; we will have to cope with throughout our lives. Depending on what we know about ourselves or what preventative remedies we incorporate in our chosen life style, we can take a degree of control in damage limitation so we tip the balance in favour of more success and happiness.

British Prime Minister, the late Sir Winston Churchill said when talking about people not noticing themselves, *"It is surprising how often people fall over something important then pick themselves up and continue without noticing what they had stumbled on."*

There are always opportunities to further develop one's knowledge to attain more understanding of how the body and mind works. During my NLP masters training I got to know a doctor who proudly said he had learnt many techniques from several alternative therapies, which enable him to feel the patient's pain intuitively. He said, this helped him to quickly get closer to treating the cause and not just the symptoms. This method of diagnosis turned out to be a sensory adaptation of intuition and telepathy. With the addition of a few coaching style questions, his patient's subconscious intelligence was describing more precisely what their symptoms really were and less as the conscious mind perceived them to be.

I deduced where possible he incorporated essentially the same non-interfering attitude as I had discovered was so important to my support healing. He was averse to any medical drugs with bad side effects requiring further medication to solve those induced problems. It became obvious to me that he was relying heavily on connecting with his patient's subconscious intelligence. I further surmised whether he realised or not, he was discretely focusing on underlying emotional issues. This inferred that where he deemed this method was appropriate, he was essentially relying on the patient's innate healing intelligence to do the real healing.

My personal experience and analysis of stress and stressors is they are actually addictive. It is not the stressors and stress that are addictive in themselves but the cortisol and adrenalin caused by stress that drives the process. Therefore, for obvious reasons as I was not so aware of this, others also may not be consciously aware of this addiction. Now ask yourself how many times you have heard of people putting up with the most terrible relationships, or working in really dangerous conditions.

This may be a fundamental reason why we feed, tolerate or indeed develop our acceptance even lust for stressful situations. A case of addiction to high stress is that of extreme sports. This is possibly demonstrated in the fact that the popularity of skiing, snowboarding, sky diving and mountain climbing are continuing to grow despite high costs and increasing deaths. Anything that is exhilarating develops a form of stress followed by adrenalin hormones and other feel-good or reward neurotransmitters.

On average forty people die a year climbing Mont-Blanc and the toll of deaths due to off-piste skiing and being run down by avalanches are also growing. Even so, the numbers of those searching for off-piste skiing are rising not falling. Skiing off high mountain peaks, involving freefalls of hundreds of feet also seems to be growing. Touching down in a burst of snow plumes on another steep slope and then skiing on without the slightest hesitation to the next big jump is superbly exhilarating if you happen to have that lunatic mindset and get a kick out of starting avalanches. People who follow this extreme sport invariably ensure they are videoed in the process. These extreme skiers get a dopamine and adrenalin kick from their sport participation also get another adrenalin kick just by watching the video of themselves. Could this be your favourite stress/adrenalin/dopamine addiction? Maybe sky diving in a wing-suit off the highest cliffs, descending at the speed of an air-to-ground missile and finally releasing a parachute to glide gently to the ground having once again cheated gravity and death. Maybe this is what supercharges your body's addictive needs. Perhaps you get your stress and adrenalin kick in some other way like stamp collecting. You laugh, oh yes; I have a hard negotiating business manager friend who gets his biggest thrills by acquiring incredibly rare stamps he has been tracking down for years. For him it is like mining gold and then hitting the mother-lode. Maybe slack line walking thousands of feet above a mountain gorge does it for you. Perhaps you are something of a masochist and deliberately provoke your manager at work who as a consequence repeats a process of mobbing you. Oh yes and there are more mind boggling hair-raising ways people get their stress/adrenalin secret thrills and dopamine rewards. This is the same reason many people watch scary movies.

The stress of winning and then completing a complex contract certainly did it for me, the greater the risk especially if dangerous, the greater the challenge. Succeeding meant a higher adrenalin/dopamine reward. Believe me, winning a legal battle in court on behalf of a client and out-manoeuvring a cleaver barrister and my opposite expert witness trying to set a trap for me to walk into; could at times produced quite an adrenalin high. Breaking the rules unmasking those who I was certain were peddling fake information as established fact could elicit a sharp rebuke from a presiding judge. Nonetheless, pulling this off in a stylish manner without any recourse to open aggression was a definite high spot for my ultra ego with its accompanying abundance of feel-good rewards.

This meant in my capacity as a business owner, I was permanently in a high stress situation and there was no room or time for anticlimax. This was because the next addictive-stress situation was already happening, plus others were crowding in for their turn. This can so easily be the life of all high performers. It all starts by constantly pushing ourselves or being pushed from those higher up management, indeed also the ever greater demands of clients. Perhaps the worst or the best is once again rising to a challenge just to prove and maintain a reputation for pulling off the seemingly impossible.

This is how what starts as a drive for success ultimately turns into the tail of success whipping the dog of invention when we most want to take a rest. In business; life is far from all successes. Imagine the stress of managing full to overflowing order books for a year ahead and then being hit by inflation rocketing to 27%. Clients fearful of rapid rates of rising costs begin cancelling their orders like falling autumn leaves in a chill wind despite guarantees of fixed prices. Then there are the stresses of crippling cost entailed in maintaining staff levels or having to let them go because the work has vanished in a few weeks. Beyond this there is the added stress of doing all this to faithful staff knowing new jobs are difficult to find. This latter case is raw, brutal stress. There are no feel-good hormones and neurotransmitters, just more stress and cortisol. It is like cold steel being driven into vulnerable flesh, after the first penetration there is nothing that will stop the pain.

In analysing why anyone, let alone myself would put up with this situation of high stress, revealed the presence of a very addictive process. Growing a business can be risky, challenging also rewarding in many ways. There is a learning curve of risk-taking that is essential if any company is going to perform well. Business is the risk business. Nothing ventured is nothing gained. This is a very real fact in the business world.

I realised there are two types of entrepreneurs. One group understands the importance of risk. Without the risks or knowing how to manage risk, risk destroys them emotionally in the fear of failure.

With their fear driven focus on the failure prospects, it is inevitably that that is exactly what happens.

The second group know about risk management and that is where the addiction begins. The excitement of planning high risk projects while finding ways to manage those risks to a minimum has the effect of being on a sustained high, like adrenalin on steroids. Executing those projects successfully produces more highs and more adrenalin. Yes, the stresses can be considerable, unnoticed behind the highs of adrenalin is the constant production of unnecessary cortisol with nowhere to go. As far as I can find, adrenalin and dopamine does no real harm but the cortisol? That is a different story.

Only after my burnout downfall did I understand how I had been responding to a perpetual out of control feel-good factor mentality. Without realising, I was building an invisible ticking time bomb that inevitably brought my businesses and my life as I knew it at that time, no less than crashing to the ground in flames.

The repeater stress/reward syndrome is quite a complex situation, which begins before the height of the stressful event. Unpicking this mess eventually resulted in me discovering the secret to real high performance is high performance planning and preparation without the stress. Without understanding this, the adrenalin and cortisol rushes power the whole process with unstoppable reserves of energy and the excitement of superfast thinking, solutions, and endless creative thinking performance. The problem is there is no respite for recovery and that is how the downside begins.

The question is, if we take that excitement out of the equation, we also take the incentive, motivation and the reward out too. The answer to the first part of this conundrum is thinking or rather using the brain in a completely different way. Part of this strategy is learning how to think and plan with the subconscious mind where stress does not exist. The big added bonus is the subconscious mind only knows truth, therefore this style of thinking makes no mistakes. A second and vital level to this bonus is that the subconscious mind is connected to the field of energy and information. Therefore one understands aspects of risk and forward planning beyond any conscious mind thinking and that is certainly one way great swathes of stress are eliminated. No high stress means minimal unnecessary and damaging cortisol. This does not solve the problem of high performance addictive hormone feel-good rewards but at least there is no constant flow of cortisol to spoil the party. Like so many aspects of balanced life, demanding sustained high performance plus high risk has to have the right accompanying factor of subconscious intelligence. If one of them is missing then either high performance does not happen or stress and cortisol pulls it down from the inside.

Adrenalin and dopamine reward may come in the excitement of not only succeeding but also beating the old stress thinking patterns. This should result in a virtually unending "Wow effect" with all the rewards and none of the down sides. Knowing there is no attached cortisol is a double whammy bonus of immense proportions, which is the cherry on the cake. It is just a pity I did not understand all that before hitting burnout.

For the unwary, as in all other addictions, the addiction becomes the tail that wags the dog. Everything appears to go superbly well and all the time unknowingly one is heading for the cliff edge. As we approach the eventual tipping point; without this essential knowledge; we are already damaging our health, thinking and performance. Stress becomes dominant and that begins to change our attitudes, behaviours and health wellbeing from the inside out.

The actual tipping point begins where successes become fewer as stress driven mistakes begin to pile-up. As stress and cortisol increase, the excitement of chasing risk fades, as does the flow of adrenalin and dopamine rewards. Thus all one is left with is stress and buckets of unnecessary cortisol. Burnout does not just put a damn great spanner in the works of your life and career; it is also associated to triggering any number of health problems.

The down side of long hours of work does produce both mental and physical fatigue. This fatigue should normally break the stress cycle as sleep becomes essential. Those with the sense to know when enough is enough should be spared the devastation of burnout. In fact it is not that simple. In my experience and I know it is the case for other stressed business managers, nights are frequently dominated by the subconscious brain doing its best to sort out the mess of our conscious thinking and show us a better way. This means day and night merge into an endless stress cycle. Tough self leadership and soldiering on against all odds can be another form of excitement. The unseen danger is that unstoppable mental and physical energy is fed by the combination of adrenalin and cortisol. At this stage we turn into cannibals feeding off our own life force energy reserves. Eventually this process drains everything including our reserve tanks. That is when the burnout crisis strikes with unforgiving vengeance as it slams on the breaks and takes complete control of the future and everything that follows.

Our stress and survival intelligence centres were originally developed at a time when we needed added high performance adrenalin and cortisol to supercharge our muscles. The purpose was to help us to run away from or fight whatever wanted to harm or eat us. In our modern world there are fewer sabre tooth tigers yet those stress processes are still working exceedingly well and come in many forms and disguises. Now we are producing far too much cortisol and adrenalin for our body's to process properly. What has changed is in our predominantly sedentary life styles, we no longer have fighting or running for our lives to burn off excess cortisol.

When considering the heart is largely made of muscle tissue, if the heart fails because of excess cortisol for too long a period with nothing to do, well "Ooops" that is a serious problem. Going to the gym or for a jogging session may be good for our health but as far as the unnecessary cortisol and adrenalin are concerned, it is invariably too little and too late.

Burnout leads to reduced motivational impetus known as "the want to but cannot syndrome." This syndrome is the antidote to risk excitement, dopamine, adrenalin and cortisol. Disrupting capability makes all but basic forms of work or exercise simply impossible for the burnout victim to even contemplate, let alone deal with. Additional side effects are high levels of body inflammation, and weakened immune system, which means homeostasis and wellness, hit the floor like a proverbial lead balloon.

One key to understanding the principal after effect of burnout is this "want to but cannot syndrome." This is the ultimate learning experience of change behaviour. This seems to reside within or be closely associated to the subconscious Survival and Self Protection systems intelligence. This system is immensely powerful in blocking new initiative to do again anything remotely related to the behaviours or habits that led to the burnout. This is an example of how processes normally important in helping our performance can turn inwards to damage or destroy any chances of doing that.

Albeit the doctor is an important first call, other specialist therapists may be better suited to help us deal with high stress. For example; Since the standard medical answer is anti-depressants, well known for their undesirable mind-numbing and sluggish-performance thus an experienced life coach trained in advanced stress management such as Neuro-fault Protection is certain to be a better choice. Many sufferers not aware of modern methods such as life coaching may prefer to avoid the anti-depressants and live with the stress as a default solution. Just thinking about this self destructive choice of behaviour horrifies me in knowing what a vicious cycle stress really is.

Because most stress is directly related to emotional intelligence, by smothering it with anti-depressants we are ignoring both the stressor and its raison d'etre. This is how we so easily compound the underlying emotional problem, thus turning a molehill into a mountain. Ignoring a persistent problem whether medical or emotional has always been a poor or patently wrong treatment option. Remember that pills and potions mostly treat the symptoms but rarely cure the cause.

Although there is quite a list of recognised methods for reducing stress including physical exercise, self-hypnosis, yoga, side splitting laughing, and even indulging in the act of sex, at best; despite wishful thinking, they can only be short term remedies. Cortisol is intended to be burnt-up immediately in physical effort. Its purpose is to enable the lungs to suck in more air and oxygen. This is to also help the heart to pump oxygenated adrenalin and cortisol loaded blood flow harder and thus to enable leg muscles to work faster or arm muscles to fight harder. The best solution in any stress situation, which is not immediately life threatening; is to stop the stress and therefore, stop the production of unnecessary excess stress hormones before they are released.

In today's business, work, social or personal environments, fighting the boss, getting angry with irritating clients and then running for our lives to our nearest gymnasium is not smart. Doing that every time you are stressed is either anti-social, impractical to keeping your job or for many unfit people; it is possibly life threatening in itself. Because cortisol ideally needs to be used up immediately in muscle exertion, the only truly valid solution is to neutralise the stressor or cause at source. This adrenal gland wonder kit of pre-historic survival sits happily perched on top of the kidneys. As one of the kidney's other purposes is to clean the blood, the two lobes of the adrenal gland are in a perfect place to get their hormones directly into the blood stream, already on its way to feed muscles at lightning speed. The key to preventing this from happening is to develop modern performance strategies powered by the lightening speed of the mind to protect itself. This is done by programming the subconscious mind to spot a rising stressor long before there is any conscious awareness of being stressed and directing the stressor behind a virtual stress barrier before it does its damage.

DEALING WITH TRAUMAS

Medical experts advise in their books, research papers, websites and weblogs that traumas (emotional stress) are a major cause of concern as they are often an emotional jolt to the immune system. A sudden trauma as mentioned above, can tip the emotional system over the edge of survival. When a household electrical circuit is overloaded it either trips the safety switch, burns out a fuse or sets light to one or more of its component parts or connecting wires. That is roughly what and how excessive levels of traumas, stress and cortisol do to the brain and body.

Consider the following scenario of a physical and mechanical process of how overloading has equivalent effects as cortisol (inner fire). Certain hover boards and mobile telephones came into the news as susceptible to bursting into flames. The cause of the problem was traced to the internal stress of rapid battery recharging. Strange to say this also applies to us humans. When both our mental and physical energy batteries are running on empty with barely a chance to rest, relax and recharge, we stress our entire system. It could be said we begin to heat-up or as the saying goes, we begin to get hot under the collar. But if we push ourselves on regardless we have to draw energy from somewhere. The problem is then the system is effectively heavily overloaded in respect of workload relative to available mental and physical energy that is the tipping point when stress rises sharply and the body produces excessive amounts of cortisol. Eventually something has to give, catch fire and given enough repetition, burnout.

Unlike mobile telephones, our survival and self protection and inner healing intelligence centres are monitoring the fact that levels of damage are reaching dangerous limits. My conclusions are that part of the burnout process is this inner intelligence's strategy to stop further brain and muscle cell damage. This intelligence understands that to halt all stress situations will stop the unnecessary production of cortisol. On its own, the only way it can do this effectively, is to shut down the entire system. In effect it is our survival, self protection intelligence saying; *"it is taking unilateral action to stop us in our track.* As Tim Spector says, *"before we kill ourselves too early."*

In this event our inner healer is shutting down our ability to work, worry, be effected by stressors or even think cohesively about anything. If our mobile phone burns out, we buy a new one. Unfortunately where brains are concerned, we do not have that option. The upside for us is that given time and the right support the brain can repair and rebuild itself. Thus the following burnout event crisis is a purposeful psychological survival self-protection process. The process is as though our inner Fire Brigade has shut down the cause of the fire, plus all but basic operating systems. The result is we are incapable of working therefore we are effectively pulled out of any further stress situations at least for the near future. Because the brain has the capability to regenerate itself, it is able to ensure we have a rest to restore our systems also to give us time to reflect on the root cause and decide how to change our not so clever life and performance behaviours. As far as the right support is concerned, this all depends on contact with the right experts to advise and guide us. This process is learning new mind skills in order to build new brain thinking pathways but this may only begin when our Survival and self protection intelligence permits.

There are no options, we are forced to stop and reflect. Of course this works in slightly different ways for different people also relative to the degree of stress and burnout damage. As we try to recover and get back to work we begin to discover the "want to but cannot syndrome." It keeps us out of more trouble as the first thing we attempt to do is go straight back to what we were doing before.

In my own case, as there was little available support or knowledge at that time of what burnout was and how it affected me, my self-healing started by finding as much about it as I could. The mass of information as we know it today did not exist at that time. Therefore my efforts were directed to the occasional research program with the addition of continued self analysis. Today there are many books and a great deal of information about burnout on the internet, although much of it makes me want to cringe, as most of the advice is naive and born out of old school redundant psychology beliefs and largely the blind leading the blind.

This new learning curve in the midst of burnout was quite a challenge in its own right. While occasionally I experienced some stress, on the whole I was running on auto-pilot (intuitive thinking). During the subsequent analysis stage, I found it interesting that even to start with, "the want to but cannot syndrome" did not stop this new study activity. Later, as I learnt more about how this syndrome works, it became apparent that anything that supports the healing process gets a green light. Anything that harks back to the past definitely gets a red card and kicked off the field of play.

This turn of events proved particularly interesting with reference to finding the most appropriate occupation in life with the least unnecessary stress. The fascinating take-away is that our choice of occupation may be doing the right thing in the early days. What is not so obvious is that every profession has its appropriate shelf life according to personal and professional development, also dare I say, destiny. Then it is time for us to take notice of the proverbial writing on the wall of our intuitive intelligence and move on as indicated. This can mean changing job, changing employers or promotion. What few realise is that maintaining a balance may include switching careers. Today, it is quite common to have several careers, preferably one after the other. This is particularly valuable for high performers in preparing themselves for the really top jobs. For many people, miss handling an opportunity may lead to being stuck in a going nowhere job that may build considerable subliminal and peripheral stress.

When understanding this process, I recognised that is exactly what had happened to me about two years before my burnout. I did recognise at the time the enormous stress was taking its toll on my life. I did make efforts to get out. Unfortunately, owning several companies is not like being an employee and picking up sticks and moving elsewhere. Finding buyers even during shrinking inflation and improved business turnover did not help the exit process. In view of this situation I opted for a half way solution of changing my work patterns. These changes did make a difference. Not understanding or being aware of the underlying process of disconnecting, one set of my stressors that had been neutralised by this change were inevitably taken over by new stressors. This was because I had not made the necessary full disconnect. In short, at that time I did not understand the mechanics of overwhelming stress, therefore, I had not done enough in the direction of radical change and thus paid the price of more stress fudging this important stage of my life.

Although pure conjecture, because there is only circumstantial evidence, the outcome has been that burnout did what I had not been able to do under my own steam with rational thinking. The result was those companies that had not failed during my burnout allowed to fold. This was the worst of all circumstances for me. Finally my last company a mere shadow of its former self was sold and I completed the separation of my old life to start a new one but what a price I had paid in the process. Then I found myself i a no-man's-land, neither fish nor fowl or any idea what was to come next.

My first hurdle was in understanding my addictive need to get back into that old business creating stress. This was manifest in my relentless effort to fight against this self protective blocking device preventing progress as I wanted it to be. The awareness of this blocking intelligence simply incited a desire within me to find how to overcome it. My persistent efforts were possibly getting me too close to achieving this for my own good. That is when that awareness of the "want to but cannot syndrome" changed its form. One day I woke up to the perception of an impenetrable wall directly in front of me. This was a very clear sign blocking my way forward. This virtual wall was impossible to breakthrough, climb over, manoeuvre around or tunnel beneath by any means.

Despite this, my addictive entrepreneurial drive was so strong that I continued to spend my time and energy looking for how I could defeat the wall. Eventually, exhausted, demoralised and completely lost in where my life was going, I stood back and accepted I had better turn in another direction where there were no walls blocking my path. The next thing I said to my personal puppet master was: *"Okay, I get the message that I am going nowhere until I have learnt precisely what I have done to cause the creation of this wall and actually change everything I am currently aiming for, which you consider is patently not in my best interests."* What happened next was the intuitive formulation of a plan that would take me right out of my existing environment and true to my Viking heritage, burning my boats so there was no way back.

Having been through all these amazing twists and turns of my "Survival and Self Protection," the "want to but cannot syndromes," and my "protector wall," I began to emerge out the other side of burnout. I now have considerable experience of exploring every conceivable nook and cranny of this modern ailment. I feel confident in saying, "the want to but cannot syndrome" is a very real problem for all victims of burnout but for all the reasons I have touched on, it is essential. This can also happen in the burnout run-up process of "stress overwhelm," this half-way-house is often mistakenly believed to be burnout proper. Looking back I realise I had reached the overwhelming stress, half-way-house when I first tried to exit my companies. Failing to do that took me on the definitive and final road to full burnout.

In the early stages I found the moment I tried to get back to work, the force of this syndrome intelligence simply knocked me out of court in no uncertain terms. This was in the form of dramatic all encompassing exhaustion that left me incapable of anything but the most basic survival activities of sleeping, eating and a minimal amount of physical exercise. In the early stages of burnout, even reading a newspaper or watching television proved exhausting.

When not left wasted, I had little to do but monitor my slow but steady forward progress and plan my next sortie to break out of my invisible gaoler's iron grip. If I pushed this process too hard or too fast, I was inevitably slapped back in no uncertain way with unbelievable fatigue. I suspect this was caused by the associated intelligence as I have observed as the 7th Sense Survival and Self Protection intelligence noted to occur in cases of devastating trauma.

Survival is by definition a process to survive a trauma and then move forward to a new normality without the stress. The danger is that people may get stuck in a mental survival mode so survival thinking and associated behaviours become a way of life. This is quite apparent in the case of alcoholics and druggies who having lost everything, they suffer their own form of burnout. They live in cardboard boxes in the streets, under bridges or in abandoned buildings. They are stuck in that state to the extent they are hardly able to even think of progressing forward out of that situation. The fears and stresses of moving forward are then far greater than the stresses of the very basic survival as a way of life.

Moving out of and away from the direct effects of burnout had changed so much of my thinking behaviours. My experience of understanding how support healing worked, certainly helped me heal myself. Paradoxically, I only began to make good progress when I learnt to stop interfering with what I thought I had to do to get back to business. A large part of this healing and change process was learning about the immense power of the subconscious mind and how to work with it not against it.

Clearly modern performance strategies free of stress are needed in a highly stressful 21st century. In this life we have completely out grown the slow pace of evolutionary thinking development through prehistory. In my book, "High Performance After Burnout." I explain new strategies to deal with burnout and damaging stress by creating purpose designed subconscious performance strategies and virtual stress barriers.

Though burnout brings normal active life to a sudden standstill for a considerable period of time, some people see it afterwards as an important major lesson in reorganising their life. Given the nature and brutality of the process and losing all I had built over more than twenty five years, I am reluctantly inclined to agree even though almost twenty years later and reading my intuitive or sensory writing on the wall, I still have my focus on better and greater things for my future.

It has been a long road to learn so much and creating a new future. Depending what comes out of my effort and research, only when I get more out of the process than I lost, will I be able to make a valid judgement as to whether it has been a truly fulfilling journey.

Dr Dina Glouberman in her book "The Joy of Burnout" writes how burnout unlocked the way to a better, brighter future for her. Provided with a good understanding, supportive family and adequate financial resources, travelling this life changing drama and retraining for a new profession may be challenging but hopefully not too painful. Anyone like myself without or with only a few of these resources may find the burnout experience less of a joy and more of another trauma, albeit; perhaps a different type of trauma. The best I can say is that whether a paradox or not, whatever we get in the burnout process and after, is most possibly exactly what we need to eventually move forward along the right track to the stage of discovering what life and destiny had really meant for us.

In my own case, long before popular gymnasiums, I had no psychological or family support, and the best the medical profession could do was recommend a holiday. As anyone knows when hit by serious illness, also the loss of a partner, wife or husband, all but one or two friends simply fade into the background. This certainly happened in my case. The slightest suggestion of me seeking moral support from my friends, I had the feeling of being sidelined as if I was highly contagious. Consequently my only option was to rely on my own resources.

My first inspiration was military training in map reading, i.e. first be certain where you are before moving in any direction. This meant I had to find for myself what sort of, and the depth of mess I was in and then worry about how to fix it. This course of events led me to making avoidable mistakes some of which proved costly. Eventually I was forced into a tenuous situation of having no idea what was coming next.

My conclusions were to do everything possible to be fully aware of myself. This led me into studying NLP, which is a very modern and effective form of psychology and psychotherapy. Then I moved to life coaching, which is another form of psychotherapy focused on performance and moving out of a stuck place. Finally I took in SportsMind coaching, which is a derivative of life coaching and NLP but focused on working with the subconscious mind to get to the highest performance possible.

All three disciplines have been important and combined they created the basis for developing MindPower Recognition and Neuro-fault Protection performance strategies. As to the up-side, this combined process helped me to be more balanced in enhancing smart thinking, forward planning and self motivation. Having got myself and my life so out of balance during the preceding thirty years, I have never worked so hard at understanding the importance of how to keep a balance.

Stress-Burnout is quite different from mental or emotional breakdown. Apart from the physical damage of years of excessive cortisol poisoning, Stress-Burnout is the mind, body/mind saying – don't abuse your mind, body and your life any more. Since you have demonstrated you are incapable of doing this, we (subconscious – inner healer – mind body/mind and other intelligence centres) are making sure you do not do that again.

A mental breakdown is an impenetrable fear and panic of life itself. In mental breakdown one simply cannot face people and life so there is no chance or possibility of the "want to but cannot syndrome," let alone the need of an impenetrable virtual wall blocking all efforts in getting back to the illusion of a normal life.

This is exactly what Dr Dina Glouberman means by unlocking the way to a better, brighter future for her. For more than two years while struggling, in my effort to restart my life, I fought to answer my absurd question, "when could a business not look like a business." This is sort of like trying to convince a failed police breathalyzer test that the alcohol was for medical reasons. This illustrates how stress distorts thinking patterns. This illustrates I was determined to get back into business and not be beaten. Hardly surprising my defence wall remained unassailable in all senses.

When not plotting how to break this colossal barrier facing me, I spent my time studying myself and anything I could that related to burnout and high performance without stress. Eventually I was writing articles for magazines and then began writing book manuscripts. My first published book was The Mind Manual. Writing held my focus and fascination to the extent I had no time to fight or even think about the wall anymore.

The wall had become part of my life but it was not until after the second or third manuscript that I realised it had vanished. Not only was the wall no longer apparent I also realised I no longer had any desire to get back into business. Despite its own problems and challenges, writing with interspersed coaching of some very special people with extra special problems, seemed to be the new way for my life to express itself. Sometime later I set up MindPower Recognition, which is more a research project rather than a company. For the time being this seems not to bother my 7th Sense Survival and Self Protection intelligence or re-invoke the "Wall" or indeed the "want to but cannot syndrome.

I mention that when we do the right thing that fits our true self, no matter what the challenges, we will find a way forward. Despite the first faltering steps, the avoidable embarrassing mistakes, the sniggers or the doubters; it seems to be natural and in many ways it flows with an ease free of distortions, major stressors or stress.

Certainly facing the challenges of learning about the mind and how my support healing worked, writing about these things helped to develop my greater understanding of these subjects. However I was not out of the woods just yet. In addition to all its other challenges, burnout had left me with an extreme form of dyslexia. I suppose, first understanding and then learning how to overcome this problem, was an early example of me putting all my learning of how the brain works into practice. Like dyslexia, every obstacle automatically turned into a new challenge and a new learning and discovery project. Although familiar with writing complex proofs of evidence as part of my earlier profession, I had never before considered writing as a way of life and was amused how it had sort of crept up on me also the fact it entailed a great deal of work and reflection, it was nevertheless, something I enjoyed doing particularly it put purpose back into my life, far better than sitting in bars, reading newspapers and watching the world go by.

Looking back there were a few markers foretelling of this turn of events although nothing about the trauma and brutality of burnout. One of those markers was being stopped in the street by a gypsy woman. This resulted in being told she could see my life being dominated by writing. Certainly this came true as my profession developed into the legalistic realms of expert witness. As my professional reputation grew, this aspect began to dominate my time.

That all stopped with the advent of burnout. I recalled this prediction, when after burnout I began writing articles on performance strategies in business but that was not to the degree of dominating my life. However having written at least ten book manuscripts with still more in the planning, writing is certainly now a dominating influence. The inference of dominating seems as though it is stressful. While reflecting on this point is when it became apparent my writing seemed to come principally from a combination of research and experience, but the writing itself clearly had a subconscious or intuitive intelligence connected to it. As I found there is no stress in the subconscious mind, the fact most of the creative work is intuitive has meant this life style has few stressors.

In the beginning of developing subconscious thinking as a purposeful process for avoiding the risks of stress and burnout, I was anxious encase it was just a mental creation without any real substance to it. For this reason I set up rigorous methods for testing these new mind strategies using myself as the test bench. Okay so I was not surprised when they worked on me but would they work for other people? The coaching of a number of people with some special problems soon proved that it worked for others too.

Developing MindPower Recognition was devoted to working largely in understanding how to interact with the subconscious brain on demand. When I realised that my writing endeavours were via subconscious and intuitive intelligence that was in itself amazing. At some stage of this development it appeared that not only was it via practice but also due to the confidence I had built in working with subconscious thinking that it became a principal modus opperendi for all aspects of my creative writing. The creativity side is mostly relevant to a series of action novels now in the sixth volume. Realising it was by intuitive intervention that so much inspiration and information flowed unendingly, was enlightening. Finding so many intuitive ideas and conclusions was frankly surprising.

Putting all this learning to activating self-healing, I concluded it is the process of the mind able to heal itself by me consciously recognising its powers and thus working with this intelligence and not against it, which made such a difference. I am nonetheless reminded to take adequate breaks during the day and then chill out for the weekend. This was to follow my own experiential learning and advice. I am particularly careful because I do find it addictive especially when I am involved in researching or writing something, which turns out to be really exciting.

A study released in May 2016 shows how taking breaks and holidays and having fun actually increases our life span. This can only happen by dint of improving homeostasis by improving the quality of life balance. This may be due to less stress being less wearing on inner body inflammation and all its own ramifications. Adding more feel good hormones and less stress and stress hormones will have other beneficial spinoffs. During my run-up to burnout, holidays were sidelined because firstly I was single thus no "one specific other to be concerned about" also I considered I had not the time to waste on such frivolous pursuits as they certainly would impede on my addiction to my work. Then being forced to indulge in this pastime, I have noticed how holidays do give me time for important reflection that would otherwise not happen. As these periods of getting out of my comfort zone of writing and study, reflection is important to appreciating a better alignment and balance in whatever form that may occur.

Therefore I agree the taking of regular breaks and holidays may lengthen our lives. Even so, this finding must be governed by a base line of what is a normally expected life span for each unique individual. Whatever that base line is, it must also be true in the contrary look at that research paper. This is to say pushing ourselves all the time without regular breaks and holidays may be complimentary to upsetting life balance to such a degree that any one's life expectancy is shortened relative to the base line. Given that a burnout crisis, which in the worst circumstances that can result in "the sudden death syndrome," I give particular attention to this research and revelation, thus give fair warning to others to also take careful notice.

To further enhance this uncomfortable fact of life, Daniel Goleman, PhD and Joel Gurin say in their book "Mind Body Medicine" that abnormal mental and physical stress can lead to heart attacks and sudden death." In recognising this we have to remind ourselves of the difference between effort and stress. Effort is a building process of pushing boundaries within limits of acceptable endurance and capability and then consolidation before moving forward again. Stress is a damaging process of pushing boundaries too far or/and too hard with no proper space for consolidation. When effort becomes excessive and void of reflection, it causes friction and thus becomes stressful and destructive.

The fact of a friend and fellow rowing club member dying during a race was a stark reminder of the danger of effort evolving into overwhelming stress. Whatever form it comes in, the risks are that it turns into "sudden death syndrome," which certainly comes in many forms and different names. An excess of emotional stress in the act of achieving goals, extreme physical effort, a tough training program at an age where the health risks rise exponentially to be stacked against ourselves is likely a lethal cocktail.

Young athletes notably footballers are known to drop dead on the football field in mid stride. As I am writing this I had news of the death of the former Newcastle United player. Cheick Tioté's club Beijing Enterprises confirmed that the player had fainted during a routine training session before being rushed to hospital. A press release said, "During a routine training session at 6pm today, Ivory Coast player suddenly fainted and the club immediately rushed him to hospital, but unfortunately efforts to save him failed and he passed away at 7pm."

This actually happened right in front of one of my employees. It turned out he had been playing in a local league football match one Saturday afternoon. A sudden attack on their goal meant he and a team mate had to move quickly to make their blocking defence. Patrick saw his teammate a little ahead of him literally run into the ground. Within a few minutes after resuscitation attempts had failed, the referee pronounced the player dead. As I understood the situation, even those lower league referees were trained for such events, therefore indicating these tragic cases are not uncommon.

This type of thing also occasionally happens in the top leagues despite a high state of physical fitness, well regulated diet and having regular medical checks. How many of us know someone or heard of someone fit and sporting dying following excessive and stressful physical effort. The lesson is that when we allow our lives to be so out of balance even if taking holidays; we can be playing with potentially catastrophic consequences of shortening our lives. Extreme anger can be another form of the stress tipping point, bridging stress from emotional reactions to physical consequences.

www.Medicalnewstoday.com put out a news letter from, which the following is an extraction. Quote:

"Conducted by researchers from the University of Sydney in Australia, the study also reveals that this increased risk of heart attack, or myocardial infarction (MI), lasts for 2 hours following an episode of intense anger. Our findings confirm what has been suggested in prior studies and anecdotal evidence, even in films - that episodes of intense anger can act as a trigger for a heart attack," says lead author of this latest study Dr. Thomas Buckley, of the Sydney Nursing School at the University of Sydney."

In March 2014, a study by researchers at the Harvard School of Public Health in Boston, MA, suggested anger outbursts could raise the risk of heart attack, stroke and other cardiovascular events.

Normally our internal intelligent strategies restrict potentially dangerous behaviours by causing different types of disabling pain. Pushing ourselves through difficult situations or pain barriers may seem a sign of resilient determined self-leadership. Another reality is especially after a certain age, that type of behaviour may be doing something so bad for ourselves like sudden "death syndrome," we just may not live long enough to regret it.

This danger comes in many aspects of emotional stress. Before my burnout crisis, a friend was telling me that he was being forced to retire from his London City job. Having been allowed to carry on in his position for one more year after his official retirement age all he had done was delay the inevitable.

He told me he was dreading retirement as he just did not know what he was going to do with himself. Getting up early each week day and catching the 06:45 train to London, being in the heart of the City, active in his job that made a difference to people's lives is what gave his life meaning. Having lunch with friends and then coming home on the evening train was a joy for him. Retirement meant he saw all that abruptly ending.

At that time before my own burnout, I had not realised the significance of his condition. Now I understand it was more than a joy. He was addicted to the stress of getting to the station on time to meet his friends of the past forty years on the train. He was addicted to the stress and excitement of being in that dynamic stream of high performers pouring out of Liverpool Street Station, heading to their offices in London's city centre. Recognised as one of the most exciting yet stressful cities in the world, simply by the nature of what it is, what it does and its unique energy, he was clearly addicted to his way of life and his daily shot of adrenalin and dopamine. This city layer was terrified as he had no idea how he was going to replace all that. A few months later his wife called me to say on the Saturday the first day of his actual retirement, he had gone out on his bicycle for some exercise. He had not peddled more than two hundred yards where still astride his bicycle he was found to be dead beside the road. The autopsy said he had suffered a massive heart attack and was probably dead before his body touched the ground. As he was otherwise perfectly fit, the heart attack was put down to severe emotional stress over the preceding years. As this is an example of sudden death syndrome, I regret not spotting the trap of the "addictive work syndrome," as I now realise the immense stress he had put himself under. He had set himself up to fail in the saddest way.

AN INNER INTELLIGENCE

The body/mind is the intelligence in every cell in the body. Each of the estimated 50 trillion cells is in communication with every other cell. In simple terms this inter-cellular communication is like the World Wide Web, internet or a totally integrated management system incorporating input and feedback to every part of the entire structure on a 24/7 basis.

Doctor Deepak Chopra MD explains in his book 'Quantum Healing,' how the body/mind works and how it interacts with the brain and the mind. Dr. Chopra defines this intelligence as "inner or subconscious know-how." This know-how intelligence led him to three conclusions.

Quote: "*First, that intelligence is present everywhere in our bodies. Second that our inner intelligence is far superior to any we can try to substitute from the outside. Third that intelligence is more important than the actual matter of the body, since without it, that matter would be undirected, formless, and chaotic."*

NLP MIND, BODY/MIND CONNECTION

Research has shown how the mind body/mind processes have powerful controls on our thoughts, decisions and actions both conscious and subconscious. Daniel Goleman in his book *Emotional Intelligence* argues that *"EQ"* (emotional quotient) is equal or more important than IQ (Intelligence quotient) and this is what marks people who excel in the face of life's challenges.

He says that *"Emotional competence is particularly central to leadership, a role whose essence is getting others to do their jobs more effectively because they want to and often without them noticing."*

All through this book, this is the underlying message. Our inner emotional intelligence plays a significant role in not just who we are and how we behave to the outside world, it plays a fundamental role in maintaining our entire health performance. This applies both mentally and thus physically also most importantly it manages the frequency and extent of our vitally important feel-good factor. Therefore, the better balanced we are emotionally, the better we feel, the better we perform in our health, our relationships, our professions and achieving all that we desire.

This process is further examined by J. Allen Hobson, Steven Hyman, Kay Redfield Jamison, Jerome Kagan, Eric Kandel, Joseph LeDoux, Bruce McEwen and Ester Sternberg in their book "States of Mind. New discoveries about how our brains make us who we are." For example, Kay Redfield Jamison looks at famous families over the centuries tracking programmed genetically inherited physical and behaviour patterns.

Neuro Linguistic Programming is the science of genetic programming messaging through habitual eye, face and body movements. Known over the past thirty years as simply NLP it has caused an enormous leap forward for thousands if not millions of people around the world in better knowing and understanding themselves and how they work. Since its beginnings it has evolved in various directions, one of which is used by the police and customs officials as a quick indicator of someone lying or hiding something.

The proper study of NLP and subsequently life coaching opens up tremendous advantages in greater understanding of who we are, better understanding of our family, friends, work colleagues, clients or sporting competitors and how they are processing their own unique view of the world. That is to say, what meaning words, feelings, environments and emotions have and how these things are uniquely important to each one of us. With this knowledge, we avoid stepping on each other's sensitivities. This means we understand how to communicate better with each other. The better we communicate the more likely we are at getting what we want. The result is greater satisfaction, better performance at being ourselves and therefore less stress in our lives. Because NLP gives conscious insights into subconscious emotional intelligence and awareness, a person is better able to deal with another's emotional constraints or problems. One importance of this is to prevent hurt emotions from becoming destructive barriers and dangerous emotions.

Another issue is where emotions are buried because we are unable to recognise or deal with them properly. Like unnecessary cortisol being toxic to cells with nothing to do and nowhere to go; buried emotions become corrosive and toxic to our inner balance. We may not recognise them or believe we cannot or choose not to handle them. Then those emotions become buried either by purposeful intention or accidental default. Therefore those emotional energies do the only thing possible and turn inwards. At this point they metamorphose into destructive emotional instability. This leaves us with an inner feeling equivalent to a permanent state of walking on egg shells or black ice. Thus, the basis we depend on to give us stability and traction to move forward with surety and efficiency is no longer dependable. What is apparently solid is clearly unsafe and treacherous. Thus, we lose our sense of confidence and capability. Emotionally floundering in this perilous state is exactly the same feeling one experiences when entering overwhelming stress. This is certainly what I experienced in the months running up to and for several years after my burnout crisis. This devastating loss of confidence and thus capability is the destructive force that undercut my continuing ability to manage my companies, continue my professional responsibilities or make any meaningful plans. This instability manifests itself in varying degrees of unnecessary behaviours, emotional defence barriers also other psychosomatic health issues. These consequences are simply the mind, body/mind shouting at us to stop doing something that is limiting us, therefore to stop avoiding important issues.

In understanding these issues it should become more obvious why and how innate intelligent centres take control by triggering defence systems such as "Survival and self Protection," "Want to but cannot" and other self-protecting syndromes, I have already referred to or will expand upon later.

Using this knowledge clients benefiting of NLP and life coaching therapy have the chance to revisit hidden emotional issues that morph into blocked states of not being able to move forward in their personal life or profession. Once those emotional blockages have been recognised, they can be safely released. In so doing the client may heal themselves of issues that had been troubling them for many years. Releasing emotional blockages is evident in itself an important matter. Buried emotional blockages known as emotional baggage; can be a heavy weight we carry around until eventually depleting our energy and success behaviours. By unloading this unnecessary baggage, which we do not need, it is not just life that becomes so much easier; our entire inner systems are emboldened to work so much better.

When it comes to any source of healing and self-healing, I cannot repeat this fact often enough that all centres of intelligence and information within your body, mind, body/mind are there for important reasons. Traditional Chinese medicine including various forms of herbal medicine, acupuncture, massage (Tui na), exercise (qigong), and dietary therapy experts realised this over two thousand years ago. Therefore the principle reasons for respecting our internal intelligence are to work with them, thus helping them to keep us fit and healthy.

The maxim "healthy mind in a healthy body" is attributed to a Greek mathematician Thales of Miletus born sometime before 620 BC. The reason for the saying is not clear; however about 200BC the Romans used the term, "mens sana in corpore sano" usually translated as "a healthy mind in a healthy body," especially used concerning the achievement of athletic prowess. The reason that high performing modern sports mind coaching pays a great deal of attention to not just a healthy mind but using it in the best way possible is so not to interfere. Hidden performance and emotional stumbling blocks were understood not only in athletics by the Romans and Greeks but also war tactics far earlier than two thousand years ago. Those early methods of focusing the subconscious mind so the conscious did not interfere, demonstrates there is very little that is truly new.

As I see so many modern gymnasiums popping up like mushrooms in my city, I am inclined to believe "a healthy mind in a healthy body," has been turned about. We may believe by going to the gym regularly or following our favourite sport or exercise we are keeping ourselves fit but who is keeping their minds fit. In a healthy body will they achieve a healthy mind? Is anyone really bothered about a healthy mind or truly understands what it means?

Maybe that is why so many people willingly beat themselves to a pulp on some bizarre contraptions many resembling torture machines or those designed for slave labour of the middle ages albeit somewhat shinier. Other than for the dictates of professional sports performance it is hardly surprising, this activity has an uncanny habit of losing its appeal usually within less than three months. Participants may improve their physical fitness; question mark; but the evidence seems not to manifest a healthy mind. This is apparent when I see people after a workout heading for an unhealthy hamburger bar and drinking high sugar sodas. Temporally oblivious of the fact they get a double lousy deal and the gym owners go laughing to the bank for the next nine months. The first bad deal regardless of any promotional offers is three months membership for the price of a full year. The second bad deal is that gymnasium workouts can easily be doing more harm than good. Furthermore, we all know about the weight loss yo-yo effect, so there is a big question mark about what has happened to the healthy mind part of the equation.

I will leave the true experts to explain why many of those complex machines can cause as many muscle weaknesses and resulting vulnerabilities when they are supposed to create strengths. The wisdom of this is in the knowledge that top physical coaches prefer to keep their exercises as close as possible to the body's natural movements. This is to say, many work-out machines cause the user to develop some decidedly unnatural movements that result in unbalanced muscle development.

The ancient Greeks told us not to heed the will of the masses but rather know ourselves. Like our modern gleaming exercise machines that ancient torturers could only have dreamed about, the masses are seduced into taking their eyes off the ball of what is really smart thinking. A lack of seriousness and understanding about how our bodies work and what those machines are supposed to do for us, turns into a mass deception the eye and therefore the brain does not see. This is somewhat like the thimble and pea game of "cherchez la femme." We keep on chasing fruitless games in the hope of winning. The trick of the game is to break the watcher's focused concentration and it still works remarkably well. Perhaps the ancient Greeks worked out that we make most mistakes when we are distracted by self imposed self delusion.

Talking of distraction and mistakes, it is strange to say that I had a painful albeit enlightening insight into the power of my body's capability to not simply heal itself but actually rebuild from its DNA blueprint. One day being distracted and a momentary loss of concentration I had managed to mangle three or four centimetres of one of my fingers on the blade of a circular saw. One would think this injury was well beyond the scope of self-support-healing. Although a tad annoyed with myself, intuitively I was not nearly as worried as the hospital doctor who did her best in sewing the remaining pieces of my finger back together again.

Certainly it was an instant shock and sore but as Dr Deepak Chopra says, the innate healing system has a natural ability to produce its own opiates, endorphins or pain killers and heal itself. Given my quick reactions in wrapping the wound in tissues to prevent loss of blood and soon after dowsing the wound with iodine followed by more appropriate first aid dressings, there was ultimately remarkably little pain. This first stage was over relatively quickly given the damage. Feeling in good enough shape I then drove myself to the nearest hospital. During the thirty minute drive the effects of adrenalin caused by the shock of the accident began to wear-off. My innate healing intelligence was then producing adrenalin, cortisol and inner body inflammation, hormones and neurotransmitters all part of my survival and self protection intelligence, with the result of me feeling light-headed.

The young hospital doctor kept complaining while stitching my finger together again. She told me; as if I had not noticed; my finger was badly mutilated and that when it had healed it would need corrective surgery. I put my trust in the hospital doctor and the prescribed antibiotics and followed my well practiced anecdote of not traumatising myself, "I will cross that bridge when I get to it."

I accepted the damage was bad but I knew under normally circumstances I heal very quickly. I had good after care treatment so I saw no reason to worry in any event what was done was done. Later as the horrible messy stage turned into evident healing, I did have some scaring and a degree of deformity. Fortunately that only lasted for a while as my innate healing system intelligence continued with the healing. After medical assistance had ended the doctor's words still ringing in my ears, "come back in twelve months and we will see what can be done to correct the deformity." Today, several years later with no corrective surgery, I can just make out feint signs of scaring. In fact the finger has restored itself so well it is difficult to detect which finger on which hand had been injured. Considering the mess my finger had been in, I regard this as quite remarkable. I do not believe this is some spiritual healing miracle, rather just one more example of the incredible intelligence of my innate healing systems ability to follow its original DNA or blueprint plan. All it needed was the initial medical support and then be left to its own devices requiring no further interference. Let's not get carried away by a minor finger injury. In severe cases of accident mutilation, expert medical reconstruction is necessary and important for practical, physical, visual and emotional reasons.

To illustrate the body really does know what it is doing, Dr. Cynthia Illingworth at the Sheffield Children's Hospital, UK, noticed in the case of some children, accidentally lost finger tips would grow back just by doing nothing and letting the body heal itself. One presumes this action nonetheless included appropriate medical dressing and that the good doctor was referring to there being no need for corrective surgery. By 1974 Illingworth had documented hundreds of cases of naturally regenerated fingers in children. How is that for non-interference on a considerable scale?

Although this same process of regeneration has been recorded in adults; she says it is rarer. Due to the speed of the saw blade my finger was missing a few chips of bone, pieces of flesh, muscle, blood vessels, nerves and skin. Despite these injuries my healing system and its intelligence was perfectly capable of restoring every detail presumably including my original finger print. This accident turned out to be one of so many personal experiences that illustrate how incredible the innate healing systems and their intelligence really are.

Notice I mentioned earlier that Dr Andrew Veil uses the words, *"you have to heal yourself."* That is what this book is all about. This puts the support healer in much the same category as doctors. Certainly the innate healing intelligence can do a great job by its own devices but let us not forget the value of antibiotics.

Dr Deepak Chopra says, the body can do anything the pharmaceutical companies can but so much better. That may be true even so I am not sure my body is quite up to producing the powerful antibiotics that helped my finger to heal and am glad not to have needed to prove it could. Both Dr. Weil and Dr. Chopra cite a number of amazing cases where after the doctors had done all they could, nevertheless fearing for the worst. The patients returned months later completely healed, thus perhaps proving my worst fears for my finger healing were wrong whereas my findings of the power of the innate healing intelligence capability are well founded particularly when there is no interference. It appears in those cases their patients were not prepared to be taken by the doctors limiting beliefs. Healing cancers and open wounds are certainly two quite separate issues with different problems. To be quite honest, if I had any conscious part in my finger healing so perfectly, it was because I had the antibiotics and regular change of dressings and therefore confidence. For these reasons I did not worry. Without that support, my pragmatic reasoning says the outcome might have been quite different.

In this case if there had been interference it would have likely first of all been worry stress, negatively impacting my innate healing system. Second might have been the stress of imagining the worst outcome and as I explained that is just as likely to get in the way of natural healing. The third possible interference could have been trying to directly heal myself by mind power. That might have been the worst interference of all by blocking my natural healing process. Who knows what that could have led to. Of course there is no evidence of any of this. The proof of the pudding was in letting go, letting the medical profession do their job of keeping the wound clean and safe from infection. I am certain this confidence in the combined process was all the support my innate healing system needed to get on with the work of healing. If you remember earlier I mentioned a surgeon who spoke telepathically to his patients that he had completed the mechanics from then on it was their job to do the healing.

I have mentioned already that orthodox medical knowledge is familiar with the overall health potential being controlled by inherited gene programs. Many years ago this was considered to be an absolute unchangeable blueprint. Today neuroscientists understand that small blueprint details are being updated constantly. Though not yet mainstream, more serious medical and neuroscience intervention is already possible to change gene and chromosome information to eradicate undesirable genetic errors such as hereditary diseases. One eventual outcome to this capability becoming more practiced is the concern for playing God and the potential of creating designer babies and all that that implies.

In the case of more developed states of external corrective surgery; visible changes notably to the face are the most common. However, consequential emotional and psychological changes are prone to occur. Even though the changes are what are desired, sometimes emotions need time and external support to help both the conscious and the subconscious to align with the new physical reality.

Dr. Paul Howard is Board Certified by the American Board of Plastic Surgery. What he says in response to the question of corrective surgery changing genetic codes, is this.

"Although, people who have had operations like rhinoplasty (surgery on the nose) many years before they get pregnant are frequently quietly disappointed that their children's noses aren't as attractive as their parents. The phenomenon is that people, over the course of time, tend to internalize their surgeries forgetting they ever occurred and answering in the negative to the question "have you ever had surgery?"

The National Center for Biotechnology Information, U.S. National Library of Medicine 8600 Rockville Pike, Bethesda MD, 20894 USA (Bethesda) says in a paper;

"Likewise, the results of basic research inform and stimulate research into human disease. For example, the development of recombinant DNA techniques (A form of DNA produced by combining genetic material from two or more different sources by *means* of genetic engineering.) *rapidly transformed the study of human genetics, ultimately allowing scientists to study the detailed structure and functions of individual human genes, as well as to manipulate these genes in a variety of previously unimaginable ways."*

Dr. Paul Howard says, *"No it does not."* A question is this; do his beliefs refer to the next generation or future generations? This is because the US National Center for Biotechnology Information says; *genes may change in a variety of previously unimaginable ways.* This is also referred to in Anne Ancelin Schützberger's book The Ancestor Syndrome and Tim Spector's book Your Genes Unzipped.

What I do know is that every change of behaviour has consequences. I know nothing so powerful as the human brain and its innate intelligence. It is clear that when the brain, mind, body/mind make changes, those changes are recorded and stored. Changes may be made by choice, by default, by force and by stress and trauma. To prove this for some unknown reason this innate intelligence leaves markers on and within our bodies.

Some years ago I needed to visit an ophthalmologist to have a tiny shard of plastic taken from my right eye, having been blown there in a sudden gust of wind. The ophthalmologist was clearly passionate about his work and proceeded to tell me about the timing of accidents during my life. As he was absolutely right, I asked him how he could know so much about me. He explained that each accident or related emotional trauma, even though I may not have recognised them as such, each was marked on my irises. A similar event happened when I had an MIR scan after a substantial fall when a new building structure I was standing on collapsed. The hospital doctor showed me the consequential indicators of all the sports and other accidents I had had in my life, including those caused by the trauma of burnout. What surprised me most was how he was able to indicate the approximate date and the type of each accident or trauma. His answer was that it was similar to counting tree rings. As tree rings differ according to changes in rainfall and periods of drought, scientists are able to decipher those differences as representing weather and environmental changes. The indicators on my spinal column changed according to certain types of accidents or traumas like car crashes, serious life shocks as break up of an important relationship, divorce, etc.

My conclusion is that if my body intelligence has the capability to leave markers on my spinal column and irises, then there are almost certainly markers left on my gene coding. If that is the case, I am curious to know what the long term genetic affects of these markers are. Those I may never know but what is clear is that in one way or another we are unknowingly responsible for changing our own DNA coding.

Mostly this is due to accidents and traumas but possibly also by significant events of great joy and happiness. Perhaps also in being part of a fight or struggle and being present at the victory celebration. Alternatively after years of study finally receiving academic acclaim, these are great emotional moments. Much of those emotions may be internalised and that is how genes will be changed. When those changes happen before parenting occurs, those changes impact new lives. Therefore, I wonder what inherent stresses had I adopted from my parents? For example the traumatic family rupture suffered by my mother in her early twenties between her parents, sisters and brothers all caused by an interfering busybody spreading malicious lies.

What about the traumas inherited from my father especially the highly stressful and traumatic fighting at Ypres in Belgium and later the Somme battle in France, and other WWI battles he took part in. Indeed also his WWII military duties before I was born. Only many years after his death, was I to learn how he had actually been emotionally marked by those traumatic events like a shrapnel bomb exploding above his command tent and a fellow officer being sliced in half by a large section of the bomb casing. He had been through and seen some terrible horrors of war but seeing his friend killed in such a way and right beside him must give a very special meaning to, "there for the grace of God go I." Like most soldiers of those periods, I never heard him speak of his war experiences I only heard them second had from my mother, even then, those were rare occasions. I cannot help wondering if those and other stresses stack up with my own stressors. Did my father's war time stressors have something to do with my subconscious need to take on seemingly impossible challenges in my businesses? Could they have eventually created greater problems doing what I did for reasons I have no means of ever understanding, no matter how hard I try. If this is so, what about other ancestors on both sides of my family who fought their own battles?

Chapter 14

TAKING BACK RESPONSIBILITY

Emotional intelligence is perhaps the most powerful of all thinking, conscious, subconscious and spontaneous processes we have. We are what we think because of our DNA programming is indelibly imposed upon emotional intelligence, which dominates practically all conscious thinking behaviours. Emotional intelligence is the driver of everything we think, say and do because it appropriates levels of importance to our personal, social, environmental, indeed justice and fairness values. It is therefore hardly surprising that mastering emotional intelligence has been found to be so important in leadership. Each one of us is the ultimate leader of ourselves. Although we may not be consciously aware of this fact; it is clearly important for us all to learn about and understand the power of emotional intelligence. The more we are aware of this fact, the more we are encouraged to take the best advice possible in developing ourselves and aspirations in order that we make the most of all our innate potential. Most important is avoiding creating unnecessary emotional stumbling blocks for ourselves over and above those inherent in our genes.

We may think we vote at elections with our heads. Political allegiances may seem to be based on hard and fast facts. In reality they are based on preferences, in turn controlled by emotions. Therefore, like it or not, any vote is swayed by substantial emotional content. This ultimately controls the fact we mostly vote by our feelings and values therefore we vote with our emotions and our hearts not our heads. Take for example the famous British Brexit referendum. Whether voting for or against: boiled down to their basics; whatever the level or breadth of intellectual reason, essentially all votes were based on a high proportion of emotional fear. This was and still remains fear of the consequences of staying in or getting out.

The City of London had a fear of leaving because Brexit threatened profits and possibly its very global existence and status. The Scots were a large part of the "remain" vote. Their fear was what happens after North Sea oil and gas runs out, like the city, their fear is about jobs and that points to their pockets. The leave group were voting for a more powerful fear that of continued loss of self determination, who has the right to enter their country, losing all sovereignty, the right to make British laws for British people and not having British law overturned by a court lost somewhere in a minor principality of Luxemburg. Do not forget the right to control their dearly beloved world leading military services and not see them merged into some none descript European Federal Union army. Yes it was winning by a short length but really there was no contest. The vote was really about British pride against City profits and of course the Scots think nothing of the united Kingdom of Great Britain only of Scotland. This says so much about English people's pride in their country and those who fought and fell for liberty. That emotional pride evolved over eons of wars and empire building adding to an already astounding history. This was the place where the industrial revolution began that led to so many great inventions. Not to forget a democracy and parliamentary system to be proud of. The people should be loathed to allow their country to be sold cheap to a mishmash of nations and unelected foreign leaders who no doubt have jalousies and other hidden agendas and no idea what being British is all about. The British Empire may be no more but with their Queen it lives on in their hearts as the emotional pride and history lives on and its emotional message must always be, woe betide any who attempt to sell Britain short. Although the younger generation may not be so aware and thus fear for an independent direction, it was the older generations with closer ties to the two world wars who fought for their national pride with their emotional will via the ballot box.

The same principle applies to our health. It is our emotions and values related to our feelings that control whether we stay in bed for another half hour and be late throughout the day or push ourselves on regardless or leap out of bed eager to get started. Therefore, it is the emotions attached to underlying values which drives our personal leadership and discipline, whether it is to get up to go to school, go to work or whatever we find tiresome. Political values are the emotional master that determines the nature of, which party is in power according to the people's feelings about a candidate and their political beliefs. Like politics, a successful company's values are tailored to correspond with the values of as many people as possible so they feel good about the company's products or services. Because values are so attached to emotions those emotions determine how we react, who we follow, with whom we share our time and on what we spend our hard earned money.

Because the brain, mind and body is so incredibly complex and because we have little idea of what we are doing to upset its balance, many health ailments believed to be real because they hurt, are in fact emotional intelligence or in medical terms, psychosomatic. This emotional intelligence has evolved to help us to understand there is something that needs our focused attention and to sort it out. Psychosomatic pain is as powerful as any physical symptom. Psychosomatic pain has the underlying power of emotional injury. This is how our innate healing intelligence, our survival and self protection and our values intelligence, alerts our conscious leadership. This is the meaning of self support shouting at us that we are ignoring something causing our emotional instability and therefore our very reason and purpose to wobble.

Evedently we are not used to recognising and treating emotional pain as we do physical pain, the body's survival intelligence converts and manifests emotional pain into appropriate physical pain.

In many senses we humans work like a washing machine does. A washing machine drum revolves around a bearing or two. Effective trouble free performance depends on the bearing keeping the machine running smoothly. If those bearings fail, the washer drum begins to wobble. If the bearing is not replaced the problem becomes critical and the drum begins to hit the side of its support frame and eventually it does more damage until the whole machine grinds to a stop.

Likewise, if something upsets our emotional bearings on which we depend for our direction, stability and smooth running, we begin to wobble internally. In expressing our feelings we use words like, feeling brittle, warn out, vulnerable, exposed, lost, having a bad day, life's unbearable or being at breaking point.

These are the emotional warning signs that we have unnatural wobbling inside. Speaking these words is at least a sign that the messages are getting through and the choice of words depicts the severity of the emotional problem. If these signals are not attended to, eventually the underlying invisible problems cause us to underperform, make abnormal noises or give off other signs indicating, our internal systems are at risk of breaking-down.

Having a break-down was an old term used for when people just could not cope with life's stresses any more. Possibly many of those were what is today called overwhelming stress or even burnout. For very obvious reasons many soldiers returning from WWI and WWII suffered break-downs often referred to as shell-shock due to enormous emotional traumas. The same applies to modern wars and soldiers returning into civilian life after serving in the Gulf war, Iraq, Afghanistan or other theatres of armed conflict and seeing their comrades being torn apart right beside them even being soaked in their blood. Walking away from all that with perhaps no more than a few minor wounds and bruises, does not mean they can walk away from the emotional memories and especially that one eternal question. Why them, why they had survived to tell a tale too painful to recount.

In the past because few really understood, so many people suffered in silence until that emotional pain turned into a physical condition or strange behaviours. This is exactly as described in the case history of "Quarry Workers." Then they would go to see a doctor. The doctor will examine the person while also asking relevant questions. The doctor may say something like, *"very good I understand the problem. I am prescribing some pills that will help clear the pain."*

The pills may be what are named from the Latin word placebo, meaning, "I shall be pleasing." The doctor does not use the word placebo because it is intended to trick the patient's mind in thinking they are really treating the pain. However, the reason placebos can be so effective is because first the doctor has listened to the patient. Second the doctor treats the patient seriously by asking questions about the pain, condition or emotional worry. Next there are two things, which happen at the emotional level. The patient feels they are being cared for. Their emotional values have been respected; therefore, provided this caring attention does resolve the emotional issue, their emotional intelligence no longer needs to cause the psychosomatic condition so the placebo or sugar pills are credited as being most efficacious.

We cannot treat ourselves with placebos because we know it is an emotional trick. If the doctor were to say, *"there is nothing wrong with your body, it is in your mind, get over it. Here you are have some sweets, now get out, you are wasting my time, I have patients with real health problems,"* we would not be happy. The main reason placebos work is due to the doctor's attentiveness in listening and asking pertinent questions. These questions go to the seat of the underlying emotional problem fulfilling emotional expectations. Many doctors distrust, emotional tricks, i.e., sugar pills or placebos for the reason that if the doctor has done their job properly there is no longer a need for them.

For this reason more and more doctors are getting themselves trained in NLP and life coaching in order to better understand the emotional aspects of treating their patients who display psychosomatic problems. This is so they the doctors perform better in supporting the patient to also perform better. The fact that doctors understand placebos can work but not always, demonstrates the quality, style and intonation of the questions is important because the questions are directed to the subconscious emotional intelligence not simply the conscious mind. These developments under the auspices of medical treatment, further illustrates the point I made above regarding the evolution of changing needs, actions and reactions.

NLP and life coaching have evolved to improve many types of performance via the need to care for emotional intelligence the way it likes to work at its best, thus fix its own issues from the inside. In addition, as I found with my support healing, NLP and life coaching have been carefully constructed so not to interfere with what the practitioners believe to be the solution for their clients. This indicates that many doctors not only recognise, they are also trusting in what Dr Deepak Chopra, Dr, Andrew Veil et al, say about the body knowing how to heal itself. Okay, but let's not forget, like the healing of my mutilated finger, physical healing works so much better with the ideal first aid and additional supporting professional medical aid notably antibiotics. I am not aware there were any emotional issues connected to my finger accident beyond annoyance at myself for that momentary loss of attention. Most of the afore mentioned case histories shed light on the fact that when there is an emotional issue involved, even the best medical treatment is not enough or even that emotional energy is sufficient to indeed defy death. In conclusion it becomes apparent that support healing first aids emotional issues so the body may heal itself on both the physical and emotional plane.

Learning about such care for emotional intelligence has been helpful in understanding and making important connections in why and how my gift of support healing has been so effective. It demonstrates how with a higher degree of the right finesse of intuitive and telepathic rapport and support is capable of making such a difference. The paradox is the finesse of no interference due to any deliberate intentions to heal, perceived to be effective. Thus, not forgetting I was invariably the last resort, therefore medical treatment had already done its best. Nonetheless inevitably emotional changes would have occurred within those people. Consequently, once I had done my part, many of my patients without realising how the healing worked, were realistically on their own path to healing themselves.

Following the above principles helps greatly to understand how highly charged emotional psychosomatic health conditions such as the case histories of "Quarry Workers, Telepathy with a Rock and The Racing Driver" actually work. However, because essentially the same process has proven so effective in many cases of cancer, this gives rise to additional specific questions.

Apart from contact with dangerous carcinogenic chemicals and radiation, it is known that many cancers may be due to such severe emotional turmoil (i.e. the washing machine wobble effect) to be sufficient to block the normal life cycle of healthy cells. It is the case of the Spanish doctor that highlights how emotional turmoil may go unnoticed by the patient. Was he a smoker, or did he eat the wrong foods, too much carcinogenic barbeque burnt offerings or suffer X-ray contamination on a grand scale due to faulty equipment or insufficient care or was he hiding from an emotional guilt for denouncing healers who were only people wanting to help others in trouble. If the wobble effect is so great, the connected trauma may well be the means by which cell senescence programs are switched off, thus leading to a cancer tumour. Did the mustard gas at Ypres, smoking too many cigarettes, the devastation at the Somme or was it the trauma sight of his friend being slayed beside him or all combined that set off my father's cancer?

At the time of "The Spanish Doctor's" healing he was remarkably calm almost serene. Did he have a guilty conscience about denouncing healers or was it simply the law that he was upholding. Whatever the cause that gradually became an issue and turned into a very heavy self recriminating baggage. Throughout his entire career he had a deep resentment for faith and spiritual healers and officially denouncing any that came to light. The fact is, resorting to what he hated and then getting his life back by what he believed to be a spiritual healer, he remorselessly criticised himself for being so terribly wrong. From the trauma of cancer he created a worse trauma due to a limiting presumption that his own medical profession had so spectacularly failed to achieve what a spiritual or alternative healer had been able to do in a few minutes.

We all have regrets and I certainly regret not explaining my beliefs of how I am certain support healing works. Somehow treating a doctor is a little intimidating, if not also the fact neither of us spoke each other's language. However, there is a silver linings to this sad case. One aspect is the indication that faith has very little to do with my support healing especially as Ninian worked very hard to persuade him to ask for my help. The conclusion is that all this is more evidence in my understanding of support healing is a medical and neuroscience issue not a spiritual one.

In his book 'Working with Emotional Intelligence' Daniel Goleman Ph.D. says

Emotional competence is central to leadership, a role whose essence is getting others to do their jobs more effectively. Interpersonal ineptitude in leaders lowers everyone's performance: It wastes time, creates acrimony, corrodes motivation and commitment. It, builds hostility and apathy. A leader's strengths or weaknesses in emotional competence can be measured in the gain or loss to the organization of the fullest talents of those they manage."

Concerning personal health and pre-emptive action we can take to support this goal; it is worth noting the body and all its systems functions much the same as Goleman indicates in the case of a company. The body is a team of not just fifty, a hundred or five thousand parts it is approximately fifty billion parts each with their guiding intelligence. In this enlarged team there are conglomerate specialised departments we refer to as organs, glands, bones and so on. Each is vital to the whole just as are each DNA performance program and centre of intelligence. When it comes to caring for our wellbeing each deserves our attention.

The important thing to ensure is that we do value and respect ourselves at every level. This particularly concerns internal centres of intelligence because that is how we can directly communicate consciously with any part of our body that may be having a bit of a wobbly moment. This communication may be undertaken in very private moments of deep meditation. If one does not understand how to set up and achieve this internal conversation there is an equally good alternative. The same may be achieved via extremely sensitive and specialised life coaching of the type I developed for my patients. Whichever the method, both add up to the same internal conversation, which nonetheless remains private to the individual. All the life coach is ever likely to understand is that internal and emotional discrepancies have been respected and released within their client.

A piece of this process of connecting mentally with any one part, indicates we are taking notice of each part of ourselves even if consciously we can only understand so little of how it all works. Understanding is not the real issue, it is in trusting ourselves to work with ourselves and our super powerful subconscious centres of intelligence. This results in positive action rather than dismissing or ignoring what is essentially a call for support when internal systems cannot cope on their own. This is because we are doing something either deliberately or inadvertently that needs to stop.

A painful knee that is ignored until it becomes serious invariably happens because we have been doing something that we should not. Lungs that are clogged up with cigarette smoke and tar, eventually fail to perform or they develop cancer tumours because they are forced into their own burnout scenario. The list of potential errors is long and the common and typical method the body centres of intelligence use to warn us that there is something wrong, are painful reoccurring symptoms. If those are ignored then the body's intelligence pulls us up to a stop. When brain/mind performance and thinking becomes over stressed, it sends messages like mind-fog, mental fatigue, headaches, migraine. These may be further enhanced by a growing number of unnecessary mistakes and poor conclusions or choices as we go about our daily life repeating what really does not work for us.

When a high performer fails to consciously connect with their emotional self, they are at great risk of making unnecessary mistakes. This state can so easily turn into one of excessive stress due to internal conflict and constantly "fire fighting" to correct unnecessary mistakes thus never getting in full control of their work, therefore driving themselves headlong into burnout. This need for self-respect goes beyond work ethics and diligence. It includes taking time out for enjoyment, emotional, mental and physical balance.

All these things are important in controlling the production and elimination of high levels of stress and therefore unnecessary cortisol and inflammation in the body. As previously mentioned this mindset of respecting oneself in its totality supports the production of endorphins, the body's principle natural "feel good" reward. If demanding continued high performance of oneself, once this circle of emotional excellence is in place, it is so important to maintain it. Care is essential to make sure the pleasurable behaviours within the circle of high performance are not easily given away in favour of extra work schedules. Certainly there will be exceptions to the rule. There are always exceptions and the rule is to make sure exceptions remain exceptions so they do not become a bad habit.

I have mentioned one thing, which occurs in the run up stages to a burnout crisis, it is a drop off of self-confidence. Many people may wonder at this term self confidence because it is something very much taken for granted. First of all high self confidence evolves from tested experience and that implicates the presence of subconscious competence. When subconscious competence is pushed aside by disrespect for what it is and how it works, then the downward slide can be fast and brutal.

I have ample evidence in the capability to work with intuitive and emotional intelligence to understand that combined they are a great if not essential supporter of high performance. Confidence may begin with a mindset such as, "if someone else can do it so can I." This is a great start but open to catastrophe if the essential information, understanding and necessary skills are not mastered before jumping in with both feet into unknown waters. Frequently the above mind set runs in parallel with autodidactic learning, which is when intuitive insights can play an important part in successful outcomes. Unsolicited winning insights are great and we must recognise that this style of knowledge or learning demands continued follow-up. Otherwise autodidactic leaning is at risk of becoming caught in a crisis because it does not have all the original back-up learning, necessary to drive conscious self-confidence. This may be less the case today as so much information has become and continues to become redundant so quickly. Therefore so long as autodidactic learning stays abreast with new developments the past may not be of any great significance. A chaotic situation is usually when the unexpected throws a spanner in the works requiring in-depth experience to find the solution. The key to continually developing this skill of self teaching is knowing oneself and building greater experience and fully immersed confidence in that knowledge.

When the circle of balance gets out of harmony with life style, this is when emotional balance moves towards its tipping point and chaos. Emotional intelligence works with the inner healing intelligence also with the survival and self protection, intuition and telepathic intelligence and therefore performance. Spontaneous healing intelligence works with all the sensory awareness centres of intelligence. So what about deep memory association intelligence, working alongside your subconscious ambition intelligence? For centres of intelligence to fully function, they have to team-work with other centres of intelligence necessary to fulfil their purpose. In so doing they support the remainder of the body and therefore the overall life purpose.

"If we do not use it we lose it." That is right; if we do not learn to recognise and use these centres of intelligence to their best capability we waste a great deal of our potential for high performance. Until recent decades this may not have been so terribly important. By default or by an intuitive awareness of these things; most people did reasonably well. Now the world is so small, so demanding and changes so fast, if we are to stay in the game without notching up unbearable stress, we have to be more aware of how to maximise ourselves without stress. It is now a fact that times and evolution indicate we just might do well to learn and use these skills more constructively. I am asked, "why do you always talk about high performance? I don't want to be a high performer." The answer is always the same, high performance is performance free of stress. True and genuine high performance is the best we can do for ourselves because it comes free of stress. High performance comes from our subconscious where there is no stress. The alternative is in suffering the consequences of higher stress due to reduced performance dominated by the conscious mind being disorientated by complex beliefs, false values of what we believe to be important. This is similar to body language and why police forces use sophisticated interrogation methods using neuro science. This is based on the fact when we lie we immediately and automatically set up a conflict between the subconscious and conscious minds. The subconscious mind cannot lie because it only knows one truth. Any conflict of subconscious truth and conscious story telling sets up specific changes in body language, particularly in respect of the eyes, mouth and facial changes, which clearly indicates our conscious is lying.

High performance by the use of subconscious intelligence automatically takes the process of inner team leadership to a much higher level. Normally our inner intelligence will perform at a given level subject to genetic programming and environmental factors such as parental guidance, education and support by significant others. What leads to a quantum leap in performance is when we develop these skill levels and let go of trying to do what we have little real understanding of. In getting this right we may prevent a great deal of stress by not getting in the way by interfering with the conscious mind in this higher intellect. Apart from any planned benefits, the additional reward is excelling with a bonus of a lot more feel-good factor. At its best it is equivalent to giving a feel-good bonus to fifty billion cells in the body. Can you imagine the experience of such a party? If not that means, more is the pity, you have never been even close to it.

One of the most powerful subconscious thinking strategies is intuitive and even telepathic thinking. Therefore it is hardly surprising these two skills should be an important aspect of support healing. For high performance seekers of all types, especially modern sports professionals, intuitive and telepathic thinking is vital for one essential reason of being so fast and always so perfect. Frankly speaking, if it was important to Albert Einstein and his genius thinking, I feel it would be worse than imprudent to ignore it.

We all use intuitive and telepathic intelligence. They are connected to how we make sense of knowing or being conscious of ourselves and what is going on around us beyond our five basic senses. In testing intuitive and telepathic intelligence, there is a much practiced experiment of focusing on a target person while for example, walking some distance behind them but not necessarily directly behind. Watch the person intently for a minute or two and they intuitively sense they are being watched. The really fascinating second reaction is they invariably look around and without any hesitation look directly at the observer's eyes. This is only possible by telepathically linking with the observer's energy flow. This is to say; when they look around they are effectively looking along the linking energy line, which naturally follows a line directly into the observers eyes. This is why there is no need to scan a wide area to find who is watching. It may be remembered that I mentioned this happening while I was watching a bent old woman in southern Portugal as we walked along a busy street. Moments after she stood up, even though others must have noticed her change of comportment and thus watching her, she spontaneously turned and looked directly into my eyes before looking forward again.

It may be interesting to observe how the 7th sense of Survival and Self Protection intelligence is also involved in this little experiment, indeed in real life. Notice how this ancient inner intelligence puts us on high alert when we sense someone or something is watching us. Wild animals use highly developed senses of sounds, smells and vibrations to detect danger. They may also use intuition and telepathy. This is especially in the case of prey animals. That is why successful hunters understand they have to be so careful to remain silent, hidden and suitably well camouflaged; even so a prey animal will remain on high alert as they respond to their intuitive warning.

Other than for the purposes of this book, the mistake of burnout is not one to shout about. It is an example of another form of

"Emotional trap," related to doing the wrong things thinking we are doing the right things. This mistake is unlikely to teach us anything worthwhile other than it was a bad mistake. The 7th Sense Survival and Self Protection intelligence will prevent us ever repeating those combined mistakes again. For the reasons already explained, be warned, if it is real burnout there is no next time. This fact is clearly evident when activating the "want to but cannot or do not want to syndrome." Burnout - already a bad mistake; is not finished with the mere trifle of stopping us in our tracks. Burnout has its own centre of intelligence and most effectively working within a powerful teamwork plan. This team's program is deliberately and purposefully highly sensitive to any activity that in anyway resembles repeating any of the mistakes.

Burnout destroys effort, capability, confidence, jobs, financial security, savings, careers, families and it even destroys dreams and hopes. This level of control may not just kill the very seed of good ideas stone dead, push it too far when there are unobserved weaknesses and it simply kills, end of story. So be clear there is no merit in making mistakes with your health, your mind or anything else that will mess up your life.

Take a lesson from a true master. Albert Einstein who said, *"Stupidity is repeating the same behaviour and expecting a different result."* Life must go on and there is a future for burnout victims. To find it one has to understand and respect the incredible intelligence of burnout and survival and self protection intelligence.

As interesting as this revelation is, it seems our 7th Sense Survival and Self Protection intelligence is already well aware of this fact. Regardless, there are many people who actually believe making mistakes and suffering all the resulting consequences, stress and unnecessary damaging cortisol is a good idea. They believe this because they have been brainwashed into thinking it is the best way to learn. They may have forgotten this is the ancient idea of learning by punishment, pain and suffering. In our modern world it is a slow, costly and dangerous method of learning. Furthermore, it mostly teaches us not to be innovative, not to be adventurous and not to challenge redundant ideas and power groups. These types of people say to me, "But look what I have learnt from burnout!" My reply is the only thing I learnt from burnout is how unnecessary and what a waste it was.

Of course there is much to be learnt but not from a superficial look at the experience. Learning only comes from deep and extensive self analysis. The evidence is that to date the costs still far out strip any benefits of understanding the mind patterns that drove why I did it. The greatest benefits to come are likely to be enjoyed by any who read and take notice of my guidance. At a crucial moment my biggest mistake was in not pursuing my instincts the first time I realised I had to let go and change. I had given scant attention to how I had been achieving success and growth and what were the distortions, the out of sight, out of mind costs in terms of the demands on my emotional and physical health. My intuitive intelligence was hammering on my inner door and at the time I was aware of it but did not understand its message or its eventual significance.

Practically everything in this and at least two other books I have written on the mind and performance have evolved from my extensive studies of my support healing and how they relate to working with and using the brain and mind in the best way possible. Certainly burnout came into that equation, in so far as all I had already learnt about the mind helped me greatly to find my own way out of that burnout mess with all its trials and tribulations.

Gradually I understood that letting go of everything that kept me a prisoner in the burnout and "want to but cannot syndrome," was the only way forward. Just as Prime Minister Teresa May understands with Brexit, as Switzerland has discovered, having one foot in the European Union and trying to have one foot out creates complications and the seedbed for conflict. It does not work because the rules for the foot that is in also control the foot that is out. I came to understand there was no merit in trying to keep one foot in my past while trying to move forward with the other. This is the proverbial millstone around ones neck and the unseen anchor holding fast on the sunken wreck of ill conceived decisions leading to poor or failed performance.

The natural instinct of a burnout victim, failed entrepreneurs, and many others, is finding themselves trapped in thinking in the wrong way and thus doing the wrong things. This invariably results in trying different ways to do again what they did before. First this illustrates how human habitual behaviour become programmed by repetition in such a way that it keeps us in the "repeater syndrome" driven by conscious incompetence. It shows that changing the superficial details is delusionary. Underneath it is the same animal with the same behaviours. The delusion is the fact we have taken our eyes off the leadership that really matters. This is subconscious, intuitive and telepathic intelligence with their aligned competences.

Once trapped in a high stress merry-go-round, it is so difficult to get out without understanding how this part of the brain works. In this way like so many others, I repeated the same business success behaviour for thirty years, believing it to be my principle success strategy. On the basis of, "if it ain't broke don't fix it," at no time had I stopped to analyse my success strategies to see if they had any weaknesses, cracks or where they might eventually appear. When it did break, I quickly realised I was unable to fix it and later on, in any event, there was no merit in fixing it because it had clearly become self-destructive.

I see the above as a warning as to how we can all go through life completely disregarding the most important subject of taking a break to step back and take stock. The irony of this lesson is that as our health collapses so goes our careers. Believing there are great lessons to be learnt from mistakes is pointless when it comes to mistakes like burnout. If anything the syndrome of "if it ain't broke don't fix it" is a stark warning. This thinking strategy may be fundamentally broken already but we simply do not realise it because it is performing reasonably well. Given all the difficulties we take that as a pat on the back. In reality, "Working reasonably well" by definition means it has some problems, which require aid and support. Therefore, unfortunately for us, the fact of "working reasonably well" may actually be like any structure that collapses under abnormal stress. Until that moment of actual failure it has been sustain a wobble we have chosen to ignore. Inevitably for a long time that has been a little too close for comfort to the edge of breaking down.

Evidently by the introduction of NLP and Life coaching into our lives we see a need to know more about knowing ourselves and how our bodies, brains and minds work. It is therefore interesting there is a growing need to understand how we can do better in a completely different way.

How many school reports say this pupil can do better? Oh dear what missed opportunities for the sake of the writer stopping with such a glib comment. As children we need guidance to grow especially if we are under performing. It does not stop there. As adults we need constant guidance or we will underperform. This is because we are more and more aware that what we are doing is not good enough and is effectively piling stress on stress. This is exactly because what we thought was working reasonably well; really was not. All too many people just like the case of the Spanish doctor, are now discovering what we have been doing for generations and decades; thinking we know what we are doing; we have actually been getting it wrong and are now unnecessarily suffering for our efforts. Perhaps this is a form of socio-political and economic mass burnout or an awareness of it being on the way to happening. This is already apparent as more and more international companies are giving their staff for mental and emotional stress

NLP principles and guide lines take a prominent place in life-coaching and its derivative specialities. Thus, it could be said that NLP and life coaching reduces the risks of making mistakes and thus leading to greater success, happiness and feeling infinitely better in ourselves without the old style stress. Knowing how to honour and harmonise our own values as well as another's beliefs, values, behaviours and everything else that is important to them is important. Not just important, it is critical to getting what we want and therefore more success in life with far less stress.

We talk of the right to free-will of choice as an absolute given in a free world but does free-will actually exist? Since we are literally governed by pre-programmed DNA, family and habitual behaviours right down to predictable thinking behaviours, thus, what is free will? When it comes to making choices and decisions, so called free-will is just as likely to be manipulated by redundant values of childhood impressions, modern mass dogma, extremist views, political correctness, governmental/educational, marketing misinformation and other distortions. All this eventually goes under the heading of default thinking. From a delivery driver to intellectuals, we rely on default habit rather than paying adequate attention to so many issues of considerable importance. So much in our lives deserves far greater thought. Frequently I see political leaders and other so called intellectuals making unbelievable mistakes that should not happen given adequate thought that should be commensurate with their level of education. We rely on default decisions for so much of our choices simply because our lives are so busy and we do not give ourselves time to think what has changed therefore what needs to change in our thinking so that we decide really what is for the best. Relying on default thinking combined with the fear of making a mistake or a fool of ourselves is why we make so many mistakes and why so many of us are wiser after the incident. We wonder why on earth we made the choices and mistakes that we did. We are governed by the illusion of thinking we knew what we were or are thinking.

All the above equally applies to knowing thyself externally as it does internally. On the basis of this reflection the two are clearly indivisibly interrelated. Thus, we understand every action; no matter how small; has untold consequences beyond our intention and imagination. This is apparent at every level of our body, mind, and health, personal, social and career performance. Knowing ourselves begins by understanding the origin of our thinking processes, what we think, why and how we think that - and are those thoughts supporting us, if so, for how long. If not what would be a better format?

Chapter 15

YOUR HEALING CODE

This is a true story about the most powerful healer, your inner healer. A story of discovery finding out why many people were healed and what prevented others from achieving the same. It is the story of over thirty five years of working with people in serious pain and all too often facing premature death. It also spans many years of travelling to foreign countries, which broadened the overall learning experience. This story is about understanding intuition, telepathic communication also that of observing the hidden meanings of feelings and emotions relative to our good health. Thus proving to be the prelude to my interest in how the mind works and high performance. This was via discovering how to communicate with my subconscious intelligence. This process underpins and controls what we have turned ourselves into. Thus who we are really and how we can help heal ourselves when things go wrong.

Medical research, modern psychology, neuroscience and physics have all played their part in understanding the process of bringing all the parts of the mind together. Chinese medicine philosophy, Greek philosophy and much more have also led to recognising how miscellaneous bits of information are somehow joined together over many millennia to give the world both helpful also misleading ideas and beliefs.

This story is also about starting a gradual, gentle and respectful process, which prepares the ground for the inner healing intelligence to function better when a glitch appears in the works. This whole discourse unravels the healing code. Just like your computer or mobile phone, your healing code is a unique process that unlocks whatever has locked up specific elements of your inner-healer, thus preventing it from functioning effectively when you want it the most. Of great importance, this account of your healing code; provided everything is working properly; is about the body's amazing ability to do what the orthodox medical profession; despite fantastic technological and intelligence resources; sometimes fail to achieve.

Practically all alternative therapies from massage to acupuncture to yoga and Qi-gong supposedly work by unblocking stagnant or stuck energy, also related stuck emotions. This may be difficult for many of us to fully understand because there is nothing to see and no apparent way of knowing if it is all true or just a myth, smoke and mirrors perpetuated for thousands of years. Is it really the case or is it another trick of the mind? Is it actually an extension of the placebo effect and therefore, we are essentially healing ourselves by showing our emotional intelligence that we are taking notice and engaged in the due process of care?

Whatever one might think of these questions it is one that is difficult to answer clearly, precisely and definitively. That is without entering into complex explanations where dexterity of words may be the sleight of hand that fools the outcome. Nevertheless, whether it is real by definition of external support healing effecting internal healing or the placebo effect tricking us into healing ourselves or a bit of both, what matters is the ultimate degree of healing. Given yoga, Qi-gong, acupuncture have been available for a very, very long time with consistently reported beneficial healing, one may take them as being fundamentally good. However the real and only test is personal discipline, experience and making up our own minds as to what really does work for us.

At an entirely serious and professional level, as previously mentioned, many western doctors are horrified by the severity of modern pharmaceutical drugs with their troubling side effects. A new breed of doctors is now focusing on information sheets for their patients also any of the general public so interested in being better informed than the standard commercial pumped out misinformation, vested interest driven dogma. One of these I read recently discussed the issue of powerful drugs to fix a particular health problem. Needles to say the drug has some seriously undesirable side effects. The info indicated that to resolve this, problem the drug companies produce another drug to fix the side effects of the first one. Then there is the problem of the side effects fixing drug having its own side effects. The story continues as if by its own spontaneous perpetual drive. The real winners are the pharmaceutical companies smiling all the way to the bank for the remaining duration of the life of each poor individual caught on their money making merry-go-round. There seems to be a disturbing underlying truth in the fact such drugs are essentially poisonous to the human body. The consequences can be that once started, stopping the treatment may be more dangerous than the original health condition. These news sheets explain there are alternative natural plant extracts with apparent no side effects and at a fraction of the cost of big pharma provided they are not blocked in the future by big corporation lobbying.

Enough is enough so these doctors along with western medical knowledge are taking more notice of the principles of natural herbal and traditional Chinese medicine. The underlying aim of this "soft medicine," which is essentially previously known as a combination of beneficial exercise and homeopathy is based on prevention as much as healing after the event. There is also a new interest in exotic plant extracts, which contain previously unknown powerful healing substances. In many cases the majority of these medications have been known to surviving tribal communities across the world for thousands of years.

You might wonder why these natural medicines have not been marketed before now. The answer is largely because big pharmaceutical companies cannot patent what nature gives freely, therefore they cannot market them at exorbitant prices to produce high profit margins. This shift of many doctors' principles is interesting as it also corresponds to the other social changes such as politics. This is because clearly the establishment's ways of manipulating us have ventured far beyond working in the peoples' favour so now the people demand change.

Nature's or homeopathic remedies when used properly mostly have few or no downside effects. While many of these substances are used as a curative, they can also be ideal as preventatives in the process of building and maintaining a good overall immune system. In this event healing any health problems is much easier and quicker. Some of these natural extracts; at moderate cost; have been claimed to fight the effects of aging, cancer, Alzheimer's and other diseases that normally rely on exorbitantly expensive big pharma drugs.

GOOD HEALTH IS KNOWING WHAT WORKS

Someone who constantly suffers from colds, flu, sore throats, backaches or similar, may want to ask themselves what are they doing or what choices are they following in their life to make their bodies vulnerable to those, illnesses, viruses or pains? What is their inner intelligence or inner healer trying to convey to them via these maladies? What is not working in their life that they know has not being working for a long time? What has been accepted as, de facto, for no other reason than their life has always been that way? This is a type of brain washing by default non-thinking. What are the emotional stumbling blocks, for which we create mental distortions to avoid or hide from them? What is the connection or the message between those emotional stumbling blocks and the persistent re-occurring or minor, mediocre or serious illnesses and the associated stress we suffer?

One of many causes of stress in people's lives is the stress arising from the fact of knowing we are being manipulated but we do not have the time or knowhow to do much about it other than grumble. This creates an underlying pervasive stress, which becomes habitual. Eventually we do not consciously notice it anymore, we simply learn the self limiting habit of putting up with it. That is until something touches a raw nerve and then our frustration and consequently our stress levels rise in a flash. In such a state rational thinking is replaced with rage and then we are at risk of losing control and doing or saying something we later regret. This is of course a question also directed towards, hurt feeling, troubled emotions, doubts, fears, other regrets, separated friends, divided families, lost dreams and the like. It may also be directed towards the reasons we know we avoid the friends, people, places and behaviours that remind us of those things we cannot cope with. We understand we are culpable in some way, thus try to hide from them by shutting those things out of our lives.

The development of neuroscience is showing us how taking back our leadership is taking control of our individual and unique healing code. The now fast evolving process in sports and management performance is exposing the enormous power of the mind available to us all. More importantly, as I have demonstrated already, we are learning how to access this intelligence and put its power to use on an hour by hour and daily basis.

Identifying our personal healing code is a matter of closely observing our life style, beliefs, values and subconscious habits. This is as much about noting carefully what works relative to any positive feel-good or other beneficial forms of positive payback as is noting what does not work.

The industrial revolution of the 19th century has seen its best days and now giving way to something different. Now is the time of a new revolution of technology, artificial intelligence, computers, robots and a higher performing human mind power rather than old fashioned muscle power and heavy industry. While millions of people are learning to progress, mostly it is progressing into more stress by depending on this IT technology. This is evident in a binding need to be constantly focused on iphones and tablets. What is largely missed is this is the time to change the way we use our brains and principally our subconscious intelligence. Without this change, the future is this modern technology simply becomes our ever more stressful whipping master as we learn to depend on technology and 'Apps' rather than subconscious intelligence, intuition and telepathy

Anyone wanting to stay ahead of this technological way of life might feel they are losing control. One sure way to stay ahead is to develop our knowledge of both options. Take notice of intuitive awareness, telepathic, and emotional intelligence to a far greater extent and also use the technology. It is not simply a case that if not we hold ourselves in the dark ages of thinking. By reason of a quantum jump into the future-present, at least one answer is in developing a better, faster and more powerful way of using the conscious and subconscious brain. One powerful answer is deliberately and purposely linking our brains with the soup of universal energy and information. Computers and robots must remain our servants rather than becoming our stressors and thus our masters. If this is not done by the technological gadgets and gismos directly, then certainly by the companies who create the technology and the all important 'Apps' without which we are rendered at a disadvantage.

The big bonus to our overall emotional feel-good balance of health is in understanding we can still be in control of our lives and destinies as far as is practically possible. In so doing, we avoid an enormous amount of unnecessary stress with all its bad consequences.

Whatever one's individual healing code, in today's fast moving world a dominating factor is stress. The new stress on the block is terrorism, robots and artificial intelligence. One example which demonstrates the lies is a large manufacturing plant that is spending $1.3 billion on retooling with new robotic technology. The CEO talking of this investment also mentioned the increase of 800 new staff. He said the company's ethos and success to date is that only people are best at creating, therefore, the robots are there to support them in the hard or repetitive work thus improving overall performance. Within those comments I recognised the deference to human creativity. For sure one thing computers and artificial intelligence will never likely achieve or challenge is intuition and telepathy. Perhaps that CEO understood that intuition and telepathy are the key stones of high performing creativity and an insight into how our world can work in a different and less stressful way.

FINDING THE ANSWERS

Ignoring this inner intelligence, subjugating ourselves willingly in becoming a victim of life and times is a powerful way to destabilise or even capsize our performing inner healing code. For this reason the whole ethos of Neuro-fault Protection is a series of mind strategies developed at MindPower Recognition to overcome redundant thinking practices.

Finding the answers why some people were healed immediately of terminal cancer or other serious conditions when modern medicine had no more answers was to become a major objective for me. Why some people were healed instantly of long and apparently untreatable pain when powerful pain killers or medications proved ineffective, was as much a puzzle to me as it is to the orthodox medical profession.

Early on in my healing career, one conclusion I came to was that each person might also respond in a different way to my support healing though for the same health condition. Although I had no idea what that difference was, this observation indicated each had their unique healing code. I further concluded that if this was true then when my healing support works spectacularly well, I had connected perfectly with those healing codes. This meant that when the healing did not work, then there was likely a disconnect between myself and the patient's healing code. The reason why could be for many reasons other than inadvertently interfering. The most likely was an incompatibility between their healing code and my own.

Perhaps 100% success rate is over optimistic, given that in nature nothing is perfect and why evolution is constantly in a process of adaptation and evolving. As my understanding of non-interference was crucial to supporting the patient's innate healing code and system, a likely answer came in the form that our superior subconscious intelligence is quite capable of reading individual codes of healing and harmonising with them. This meant that for the cases where my support healing did not work, somehow I was; albeit unintentionally; possibly interfering in that harmonising process, thus indicating the importance of intervening without interfering. This can be something as simple as inadvertently trying or wanting to be helpful.

The only apparent answer to this conundrum is in entrusting any form of intervention to our subconscious intelligence and innate healing systems.

Doing only the right things to support the healing code meant making the effort to understand another labyrinth of mind behaviours. As that seemed to be a hopeless task, the logical conclusion appeared to be in approaching the problem from the reverse direction. This was in identifying what I did that definitely worked and then refining and perfecting it but most importantly working in conjunction with the telepathic guidance of the patient's innate healing intelligence.

The answer may also be to do with emotional intelligence, which is clearly closely related with and governs the 7th Sense survival intelligence. Emotional intelligence can drive us to achieve the most amazing positive outcomes of happiness, pride and joy or the most stupid actions for, which we live with permanent regret. A survey done in the 1990s in the USA sampled one thousand women who had filed for divorce. After one year 90% deeply regretted what they had done and considered themselves worse off emotionally and in their balance of life.

When a patient's body refuses to respond to recognised orthodox medical treatment and does not change with support healing, the cause of this must be linked to exceedingly deep or stubborn emotional blocking. This raises the question as to why the body's defensive, self protecting intelligence can be so stubborn.

Like acupuncture; healing only seemed to work when whatever energy flow was blocked becomes unblocked. This is apparent in the patently obvious case histories of "The racing driver" "Quarry Workers" and "Telepathy with a Rock," to name but only three and those being immediately effective. The key to answering this question was in how best to deal with stubborn resistance intelligence by undoing or removal of whatever was feeding it. If this is valid that means the resistance is driven by a profound emotional injury.

Whatever the inevitable answer, the likelihood there is a resistance factor, further points to the patient creating their own ailment and therefore they have the power to heal it. If this is true, it is more evidence that the support healer is if anything supporting the healing of emotional intelligence so the innate healer can affect the real healing from the inside out.

Telepathy with a Rock is an extraordinary case because verbal communication was impossible; therefore it all happened by telepathy. In this case and that of the Spanish doctor and Christmas at home, these patients were capable of defying death until their respective emotional upheavals or needs had been addressed. The significance of particularly "Telepathy with a Rock," must tell us something about people in comas. Is the trauma pure mechanical damage or is it an emotional trauma? Therefore, is it like "Telepathy with a Rock" possible to telepathically communicate with their subconscious intelligence to find what the problem is and if it can be healed, how best it may be resolved?

Analysis of various patients and support healing sessions revealed that the emotional blockages were most likely resolved by the life coaching style of conversation with the patient precisely as many doctors are now teaching themselves to do. In the early days this coaching was entirely intuitive and, long before I first heard of or experienced it NLP or life coaching. When I eventually studied NLP and life coaching in 1998, I immediately made this important connection with what I was doing that worked so well. As mentioned earlier through the life coaching style of talking with my patients via their subconscious minds, I concluded that unknowingly I had likely been intuitively and telepathically connecting with their emotional intelligence and their healing code. This was in such a way that the patients were minded to unlock their emotional blockage and thus the resistance to responding to orthodox medicine or to the patient's own innate healing intelligence.

The case history of the spiritual church member who suffered stomach pains is a classic case that supports this theory. After a few moments of gently talking to her in the life coaching style, her pains disappeared. The fact it was seen to happen in just a few minutes and in front of apparently hostile witnesses; was clearly remarkable. In short, as soon as she had addressed the underlying emotional problem, there was no further need for the pain symptoms. Those had been produced by her innate healing intelligence to remind her she had an emotional blockage to sort out. This identifies her internal resistance intelligence blocking her healing code and refusing to permit healing by any method, until she did the right and only thing needed.

Reference to this example above sheds further light on the case of "Telepathy with a Rock. The unusual connection was that my support was not to heal The Rock's, i.e. John's condition but heal a resistance in his family to accept the truth they were so desperately trying to escape from. For these and many other examples I am convinced life coaching is itself a powerful support healing process. This likely is the most pertinent answer to the reasons why life coaching has become so popular and well respected principally in companies and corporations. Quite conveniently its name "Life Coaching" is connected to the resultant performance of healing emotional blockages rather than in the healing itself. It is notable that hardnosed business thinking by particularly major corporate institutions, NGOs and those with an entrepreneurial mind set have great trust in life coaching due to the immediate and tangible results. Life coaching has gained respect simply because it is so effective. Part of that worldwide recognition is because as with my support healing it generally works quickly.

This all brings me to wonder where is the difference or the join between my natural support healing gift albeit now in a developed state and that of expert or specialised life coaching. In raising these questions the answers appear to confirm my beliefs that just as anyone so minded can become a trained and qualified life coach, so anyone so minded with the appropriate training and experience may become a support healer as in my own style.

I believe the case history of "telepathy with a rock" is as close an explanation as I can possible get to the first support healing action of logging into a patient's subconscious intelligence. This is not to interfere but in order to acquire precise instruction of what is needed.

The Wow factor of this case was the realisation that having connected with "The Rock," I was there not to heal him but his family outside. They were the ones with all the emotional confusion, chaos and blockages. My final job was in following precisely "The Rock's" wishes. This led to the family getting the message almost instantly. After that they did not need me anymore so I left them to complete their own healing. I did have a telephone call from John's wife a few days later only to learn she and the family had genuinely expected me to heal him and there was still an undertone of anger I had not done that. I appreciated her emotional shock at losing her husband and also realised that family rocks apparently do not have the right to leave their place or die.

Doctors, nurses and all manner of health care therapists also fitness and life or performance coaches are essentially healers. They help others to improve their own health, fitness and professional performance by getting their patients or clients to get the best out of themselves and with least stress.

Telepathy is not so well understood or recognised as intuition is believed to be. Telepathy is mostly considered to be how we understand something about someone else not in our presence. Having worked with intuition and telepathy for many years, I am minded to believe they are intrinsically connected or variations of the same mind intelligence. Each may work independently while they also work in tandem more than realised.

While I have been explaining how support healing works, at the same time this demonstrates that everyone experiences some form or degree of telepathy on a daily basis without realising. If the case histories are not enough evidence, one striking experience of telepathy for me was being woken suddenly at two o'clock in the morning by hearing my name being called and apparently the person was in a terrifying panic. Albeit, this was within my subconscious; I woke and sat up in my bed instantly as if the person was standing in my bedroom next to my bed.

Immediately I recognised the voice as a past friend with whom I had lost contact for more than twenty years. Later that day I called this person's mother to tell her of that night's event. She dismissed my concern and told me I was just having a dream. The next day the mother called me to say her daughter had had a dreadful experience. While driving her car she was almost crushed by a speeding truck that had jumped the red lights at a busy road crossing. Apparently, she took the perfect split second action that miraculously avoided a bad accident and saved her own life.

I found the actions as described by the mother of her daughter's spontaneous driving skills particularly strange. That action to save herself was completely out of her normal character. Her mother had said she executed an extraordinary manoeuvre with abnormal confidence, which had utterly surprised her immediately after. My own knowledge of this woman was that she was an extremely gentle person given to a remarkably sensitive disposition. She was more prone to freezing in panic and certainly not given to anything so brutish, as extreme driving techniques. Her mother and I checked the time difference as her daughter was living in a far away country. We found two o'clock in the morning my time was about the time of her daughter's thankfully near miss trauma.

As to the purpose of her subconscious intelligence targeting me so forcibly, this is quite interesting. All I remember was being aware the danger was over and then I lay down and went back to sleep. The fact remains that this person may have had no conscious awareness of her subconscious alarm call. At one time we had been very close so I was possibly attuned to this woman's energy more than I realised although she had not been in my life or my conscious thoughts for many years.

In the morning realising the episode was telepathic, I nonetheless felt concerned as I had done nothing to help her or had I? Had I actually responded telepathically in a milli-second in the perfect way but as it was so instantaneous and subconscious, I had no conscious recollection of this happening. In terms of telepathy, this is not beyond the realms of possibility. In my book High Performance After Burnout, I explain in detail an experience of a personal near miss accident that should terrify me just to think about it. That is, had I not previously created for myself a high performance subconscious safe driving program to deal with precisely this type of unexpected event. Although quite remarkable on its own, in such a situation I would normally expect to have a boost of adrenalin and cortisol rushing around my body as I faced a truly life threatening situation. My heart beat rate should have risen rapidly followed by the mental reconstruction, self recriminations and a whole bunch of additional tortuous feelings and emotional anticlimax - remarkably none of this happened. My immediate conclusion was that my subconscious safe driving programmed had worked magnificently well; better than I had planned or expected.

On reflection, I fully realised it would have taken months of training with a specialist instructor to begin to master the extraordinary driving skills I demonstrated on that occasion. The most significant aspect was that I experienced no stress at all. This was especially as it was the first time such a thing happened. If anything I noticed the uncanny sensation of being so calm. Considering all that had happened during those few seconds, the positive outcome against all reasonable odds, should have caused at the very least a sense of elation. This was particularly given the impossibility of it all and the potential for unthinkable outcomes had it all gone badly wrong.

In the light of similar experiences of pre-installed high performance subconscious strategies being triggered automatically; these always resulted in the same calmness during and after tense situations. This supports the existence of subconscious competence as being the brain's superior performance intelligence at work. A further conclusion is that this is an intrinsic part of my support healing telepathic and subconscious capability. This is to say; none-interference really is a key factor in allowing the subconscious brain to work at its extreme best. I believe it is quite feasible that that woman's scream in the night may have activated a telepathic guidance within my subconscious to guide her to do exactly the right thing to avoid a dreadful accident and save her life. If the above conclusions are at all valid, the fact I was in a deep sleep, with zero possibility for conscious awareness to interfere, the entire telepathic link worked superbly well.

I accept all this is theory as there is no means of proving any of it really did happen; however it is backed up by years of experiencing similar subconscious performance. It would be no more than a romantic notion to think this woman had kept a special place for me in her secret garden of memories. On a pragmatic level I would put my money on her subconscious intelligence being connected to the universal field of energy and information (Albert Einstein) that knew I was the perfect person to guide her albeit subconsciously and half a world away? Yes, it sounds crazy but I and many other people have experienced equally and perhaps similar crazy things during our lives.

Telepathic communication is instant and has no boundaries or limits due to distance. It is like a telephone call to a far distant place as though the person was in the room with no time-lag at all. Could it also be that her subconscious intelligence was linked to the errant truck driver's behaviour before he crossed the red lights? In this case her subconscious scream calling my name for help, may have been several seconds before she was consciously aware of the truck bearing down on her. Possibly in those few seconds via telepathy she was guided by my own subconscious high performance safe driving program just as I had been many months earlier. If what she did was anything like the way I intuitively drove my car and trailer out of a certain and terrible accident, then to me it all makes sense. As a foot note to this story, I am not certain Albert Einstein was right in thinking he was lucky to happen on specific information floating in the soup of universal energy and information before anyone of his peers spotted it.

This woman woke me in the dead of night more than ten thousand miles away. Whatever she did do, the developing trauma was sufficient so she instantly slipped into a subconscious, trance or "Zone" state. In that condition; just as I had done the first time I put my subconscious performance strategies into operation; she reportedly understood exactly what to do and executed it with perfect timing. Unless she had trained and perfected those strategies weekly that feat alone is quite incredible. On this basis I believe it is possible that the information reaching Einstein via the soup of energy and information was somehow meant uniquely for him. If this theory has any validity then the attracting energy would have been the energy generated by the power of his focus for what he was working on. Just as this woman linked directly to me and the returning information was specific to her, surely by association Einstein's universal soup of energy and information discoveries were instigated by his specific need and focus.

In the days of our pre-historic ancestors, running, fighting or freezing were their principle survival strategies. In this case the woman could not run and fighting was of little use. As such I suspect she froze as her third survival strategy. The act of freezing almost certainly allowed her subconscious intelligence to take control. Once it had done that whatever information it needed from me, her implicit brain intelligence activated the perfect performance that saved her life. There was no time to think, "Oh goodness me, there is a truck about to crush me what shall I do? Er, er, er, Oh yes I'll send a telepathic message to Robert Denton, he will know what to do. It is the middle of the night for him but I am sure he will wake up." She would have been dead by this time. The facts are she was in a life and death situation, her scream woke me up and then she behaved in an unusual and remarkable manner, which saved her life. Developing this conclusion, sheds light on the importance of the telepathic link with my support healing, my patients also to the question; why me.

Sadly for any romantic souls attracted to the idea of secret garden memories and a lingering love, I am fairly certain that is unlikely also the entire process has no emotional content. This is simply practical evidence; albeit circumstantial; we are all inextricably linked to the universal soup of energy and information and thus to its pragmatic search engine of unimaginable resources and speed. It may be possible that the subconscious links we have already made with specific people during our lives, have a vital helpful element when any of us have a desperate need of a helping hand. I have no doubt that many spiritually inclined people would call this a spiritual intervention. I prefer to put my money on Albert Einstein's theories and physics of the universe.

There are many centres of intelligence in the mind just waiting to be put to work if only they are first recognised. The potential for amazingly successful safe driving programs or subconscious high performance strategies of any nature are infinite. This account and many similar events experienced by other people demonstrate the power of the mind also the unbounded potential and speed of intuitive and telepathic communication.

More information is available on these subconscious performance strategies at: neurofaultprotection@gmail.com www.neurofaultprotection.com and in my book "High Performance After Burnout."

There are horses for courses and then there are those who insist on putting the wagon before the horses. Whatever it is, never mind about learning from mistakes, it is far better to learn from successes. This is because anything taken from mistakes is indelibly linked to the energy of the mistakes. The real performers learn from successes because the energy and information contained within them has a history of success. No matter how slight remarkable or unremarkable successes are, they are infinitely more powerful especially when they are out of the norm or difficult to understand, analyse and practice. The simple reason for this is few others are prepared to make the effort to go this extra mile or two. Therefore performers with this level of motivation steel a march on the following pack trying to make a silk purse out of a pig's ear of mistakes. When we understand how a person's unique healing code works, these combined pieces of knowledge can so easily permit the same special healing to happen again, again and again.

An example of this is a line of research in genomes now focusing on building new success on earlier success by reading genes. Because reading genomes or DNA programming is so successful, some bright spark has realised that this technology can not only predict future ailments and susceptibilities, this information can pre-empt trouble. These preventive measures are aimed at a softer medical regime more aligned with homeopathy and less surgery. With far less collateral damage this is so much better than poisonous and dangerous pharmaceutical drugs with the power to stop a problem when it is in its full stride and with devastating side effects.

Chapter 16

When Stress Turns Black

An example of this occurred when a middle aged man came to me to help with his chronic depression. In the process of support-healing/coaching we both realised for all intents and purposes he displayed all the symptom of a chronic depressive. His story started as a family trauma when he was still a boy. He had become stuck in his very special form of emotional burnout as a boy. This appeared to be real but proved to be self inflicted to punish those responsible for disrupting his life. As he was not really broken, eventually he gained two doctorates also a long list of other impressive qualifications and then he held down an extremely responsible position. This all seemed remarkable for a chronic depressive; even so I was not surprised to learn his job actually enhanced his self-isolating habit thus exacerbating his state of depression, which had become a habit more than an ailment. So then the tail of the self punishment was wagging the dog.

I have not placed this case in the case histories section because it is strictly life coaching, although it contained support healing characteristics. Since depression is a delicate state of emotional stress, I turned to stress coaching rather than support healing, albeit as I have already explained, in my view the two are closely related.

During the coaching conversation Thomas brought up the subject of holidays, which he dreamed of but he just could not bring himself to organise. This and having his own house instead of living with his parents rang bells of the "want to but cannot syndrome." I asked if he might consider taking a group holiday package where he would meet and socialise with other people. As he would not know them and thus they did not know him or his condition, so long as he did not speak about it, he had a good chance of enjoying a nice holiday. His immediate response was, "who would want to go on holiday with a chronic depressive?"

Given he had completely missed the point I was clear his attention was so focused on his self image as the victim, he was inadvertently promoting his own nightmare. This illuminating stage of his coaching proved to be the key to eventually unlocking a serious emotional stumbling block of perpetuating his own analysis of an original mistake. This is one of the problems involved in learning from mistakes. The same mentality that made the original mistake is at high risk of reconfiguring the mistake so it looks different but in reality may be the same or even worse. This is one of the fundamental reasons why life coaching is so effective. Life coaching is to guide the coachee into creating new and different thinking patterns. In so doing the coachee may then address a problem they have been stuck in from a different perspective. As this is achieved, they can then find their own way out of the mistake or stuck thinking strategies.

There is a case to be made in the event of past performance issues, which highlight worthwhile characteristics that have never been exploited. Observing the characteristics of behaviours that drive the persistent memory of what is seen as limiting factors is likely to be emotional intelligence signalling that something important has been overlooked. At first we may believe some past events seen as emotionally charged cannot be changed. This is because of the belief of, "what is done is done and there is no way to turn the clock back or start afresh." This I deduced was this man's deliberate excuse for not facing what had happened in his childhood. The consequences were the clock of memory kept chiming the same time as when his dreams fell apart and he chose to enter his interminable depression. This sounds a cruel reflection but I will expand on this conclusion.

This is an example of how in general not "knowing ourselves," that is not understanding how our minds and bodies work or what the signals or sensations they send us, actually mean. Thus, we come to so many wrong conclusions or just do not take any notice at all. Just as we need to heal our physical aches, pains, hurts and other ailments, so we need to heal hurt, damaged and suffering emotions. This is because they are just as alive as our body is and they can, as previously discussed, lead to so many psychosomatic ailments, all being ably capable of slowing us down.

In principle I am against the concept that it is never too late. This is largely because it leads to false beliefs and eventual greater disillusionment, frustration, wasting of time, deep regrets and sadness. Another issue why it is so wrong is because making excuses until it is too late or at least is arguably too late, speaks a great deal about a poor self image, a lack of confidence and an inherent "want to but cannot" syndrome. Only in Hollywood is reality turned on its head for our entertainment. Life is life and too late is too late and yes there may be a silver lining in that being too late may leave space for something better or more suitable for those who cannot be on time with their planned objectives. Nonetheless there are exceptions to this rule. This is that it is never too late to heal emotional pains. This is not just healing emotions, in doing so we automatically release a changed state of perception, thinking and reasoning and that may change so many other issues including limiting perceptions of need, values, timing and capability.

Look closely and we should recognise emotionally charged limiting reasoning associated with what we believe cannot be changed. This falsely perceived limiting reality invariably blocks us within our sphere of potential capability. The real question we need to ask ourselves is, how do emotions become so damaged and how can they be healed quickly? How can we move on or has it all been an illusion in order that it is never too late to learn something important unless really it is left until it is definitely too late.

One of the principals of support healing or for that matter NLP therapy and life coaching is that the patient wants and asks for help themselves. A hostile or driven client or patient is never a good start. Fair enough Thomas did call me himself and asked for my help. I had the feeling that he was willing to give it a whirl at least to get his mother off his back. Support healing is one thing and life coaching another but all in all, I believe neither of us had any great expectations. What did eventually transpire was perhaps predictable.

This case turned into something surprising for us both. On analysis I became convinced Thomas knew exactly what he was doing in creating the illusion of his own black depression. He is highly intelligent and somehow understood that with the power of his mind he could make his world as he wanted it. This may have been to punish those he regarded as responsible for destroying his boyhood joy and dreams. The original mistake or what he did not see was how he got himself caught in his own trap. Thomas became familiar with a long list of psychologists and psychotherapists but he was so intelligent I am convinced he had duped and frustrated them all. Since his depression was in reality an illusion, they had no chance of fixing what did not exist.

On first meeting him, intuitively I understood that healing would not help him. Perhaps that was because Thomas knew he could play the same games as he had played with his psychotherapists. But, he had never experienced a life coach. The concept of not interfering in his life style or judging him in any way with open ended questions seemed to intrigue his considerable intellect. This was likely because he was not aware the coaching questions are designed to talk to his subconscious mind. Now he was defenceless, this elicited a rapid change in his attention, which visibly opened doors for further progress. It was clear to me he was intrigued by the process so was eager to play what he thought was a game of wills with me. What he did not realise was that the life coaching was setting up a game with different rules between his conscious will power and his far more powerful subconscious intelligence, which knew the real and only truth. As his coach I was a bystander outside the equation and beyond his own game strategy.

One of the creative things we all do quite naturally is to make plans for the future; Thomas pretended he just could not do that. This meant that his life appeared to be controlled by acts of spontaneity. All indications were his "want to but cannot" syndrome had reached a chronic state at an early age. Nonetheless, something did not fit because he had actually been planning and achieving his goals. I wondered how he could hold two doctorates and other challenging qualifications and not be able to plan ahead but still aim for and succeed in acquiring such diplomas. One possible answer to this riddle seemed as though it was quite appropriate to his condition in that incredible focused studying in isolation or in the silence of libraries, which he clearly enjoyed. This enabled him to escape his greatest fears of good experiences having to end and harking back to his boyhood troubled and hurtful experience. His answer was to stay in the dark and solitude and that way he could not be hurt. He clearly had pleasure in studying. Because he started a new study before the previous one came to its timely end his strategy was safe. In essence he had perfected the art of everlasting spontaneous motion yet it was too perfect. That might have been fine until the studying came to an end and he had to put all that learning to work.

Emerging from his emotional survival and self protection dungeon of studies into a real time job and contact with other bright people is when he saw the fulfilling lives his colleagues were living. Now he could see how by his own will-power he was missing out. I believe this was when his dark secret turned into real high level stress but he was caught in the teeth of his own deception. He desperately wanted to have friends but he had condemned himself to behaving in a way that made this impossible. As he was perfectly lucid about his behaviours, he accepted silence and isolation served his life style admirably but something was stirring deep down. It appeared to me that given the habit of years of focused study; he actually found pleasure having his head buried in a mountain of reference books, reports and data, also he had no need to face the world outside. Because the work load was never ending this fact did not fire up his fear of this coming to an end. He said that studying was very long term and the benefits of solitude gave him a sense of safety. This may have been true because it helped his studies eliminating all distractions but also served his deliberate illusion of being a chronic depressive. Then I asked him why he was now asking for help from a support healer/life coach when the best of psychologists had failed to help him? Given he was still living with his parents I was not surprised by his answer. He came to me by the encouragement of his parents, specifically his mother.

During this process we entered an exercise to determine how far forward he saw his future. I have experienced people with some fairly far off also limited futures but Thomas's beat them all. His perception of his future was about one inch from the end of his nose. Now I was suspicious and suspected he had picked up this strategy from previous encounters with psychologists. In addition, he claimed he looked at the world through not dark but black glasses. There could have been a very real reason for him perceiving his future and the world in this way, it suited the image he wanted to portray. Stemming from his boyhood trauma of his life being torn apart, he claimed he had become fearful of enjoying himself because happy times eventually came to an end and that reminded him of his trauma and was terribly depressing to him. Permanently looking through black lenses with zero expectation was his strategy for not seeing future possibilities and therefore not experiencing even the first glimmers of happiness. Although I recognised some serious cracks in his story, I had no idea of what was to be the outcome and little idea other than something intuitive was nagging at me. In the end it was the life coaching strategies of communicating with his subconscious intelligence, which only knows the real truth that broke the log jam.

Thomas did not confess all to me, it was his subconscious intelligence that compelled him to stop the farce. Directly after our last meeting, in one spontaneous subconscious act, he went straight to the airport instead of going back to his office. Now his genie was out of the bottle and facing him down. Just as I had experienced after my own burnout crisis, I believe it was his 7th sense of survival and self protection and his subconscious intelligence that ensured he had no chance to maintain his lie and deception any longer. This was his subconscious intelligence taking full control, thus he did exactly what he consciously claimed he could not do.

In many senses this case is very like that of John the solicitor in "When a Doctor came knocking." Although Thomas really had turned himself into a depressive, he also had many characteristics of overwhelming stress. I am not a qualified psychologist in the traditional meaning of the word but I am trained in the modern psychology of NLP and life coaching also I had years of practical experience of NLP therapy, life coaching also confidence in my intuition, telepathy and my support healing.

I had not judged whether he was truly a chronic depressive. Via the life coaching process Thomas had done that for himself. Very quickly he made surprising progress as he changed from sullen to bright and smiling even laughing. In fact the progress was so good he ditched his black lenses and his extremely short sense of the future. By the third hourly session he was well into planning not only his future house but also setting up his own business. Then came the big surprise. I should have seen it coming especially when a client in such trouble makes super rapid progress.

A couple of hours after our last session, I received an email from Thomas, he was in Geneva airport. He had grabbed a last minute plane seat to somewhere far away for a long overdue three week holiday. WOW!

Another client had done a similar thing as Thomas. She created her own depression as a way of punishing herself for something she greatly regretted. Although in a moderate state of depression, she suffered with a strong emotional issue as a result of her father suddenly dying during a period they were not talking. This woman lived in a constant state of seeing the image of her father directly in front of her throughout each day. This enduring reminder eventually drove her into not only depression but also she could so easily break down in tears for no apparent reason. The coaching was directed at guiding her to understand why her subconscious intelligence needed to create a visual image of her father. Once she worked through that process, she was able to return to normal. This is an example of how and why emotional trauma can cause some strange happenings in the mind's eye but also to the extent it becomes stuck in the detail of the trauma that causes an emotional log jam.

Chapter 17

ACTIVATING THE KEY

The day I started to use my healing gift the word got about and I was contacted by a local spiritual church leader. I explained I had no mentor or training, the healing was all intuitive. With this she insisted she had to train and guide me. I felt it was generally a good idea so went along with the offer. Prior to this intervention my healing was working extremely well. When the spiritual and faith healing aspects were introduced, I did not feel easy about many of them. Quickly I was at odds with the practices I was being taught so it is hardly surprising my performance and successes took a downward slide. Subsequently I ended the training and returned to my prior practices of what worked well. Only some years later when analysing the subconscious thinking of healing, did I come to the conclusion that the spiritualist church leader's instructions were pulling me out of subconscious quantum thinking; into conscious interfering thinking; the likes and consequences of which, I have already dealt with at some length in previous chapters.

Via my intuitive support healing I had no concept of how the healing worked. Beginning with the basic premise that healing the body is a formidable task, I therefore had no evidence I was the healer. All I had to go on was just that something I naturally possessed was triggering a positive reaction in my patients. Thus, I felt there was an arrogance in spiritual or faith healers believing they were the definitive healers, albeit supported by a host of spiritual guides with whom they claimed only they could see or communicate with. Even so, I found the experience educational to understand spiritualists' beliefs and the fact those suited certain peoples' spiritual needs. Inevitably my reputation grew as a spiritual healer regardless of my own feelings and beliefs. Most patient's did not bother to consider the issue although some patient's openly asked me if it mattered that they were not inclined to any particular spiritual or religious beliefs.

It is generally accepted that having a patient in a deep state of relaxation is important. The reasons are mainly for calming their mind. But then an instant healing with an agitated businessman that happened at the side of a busy hotel swimming pool turned even this universal belief on its head. The man was standing beside me massaging his hip for some time. I had noticed the same man the previous day doing the same thing. Watching the man I became intuitively aware the real problem was in his ankle not his hip. I asked him what the problem was. He said his foot had slipped on the edge as he had dived into the pool. He considered in so doing he had trapped a nerve. I asked him if he would like me to help him. Curious, he looked at me for a second.

"Are you a doctor or something else like that," he asked.

"Something else will do," I replied.

"Oh really, well if you think you can fix it, yes okay."

Intuitively I placed my hand on the ankle of the leg he was massaging and then squeezed firmly. The man jumped in the air with the shock of a sharp pain running up his leg. As the pain dissipated, his face changed in expression as he recognised he had no more pain.

This was not a miracle of spiritual healing driven by holy waters of Los Angeles entering my body and administering God's gift of healing, neither was it the man's or my faith. Anyone trained in acupuncture, acupressure, osteopathy any number of martial arts, even yoga, indeed anyone open to intuitive awareness could have achieved the same outcome given a little focused attention. It was clear to me that the man was right, he had trapped a nerve. By me trusting my intuitive and telepathic intelligence, I did not have to go through a detailed examination of the man's leg. Furthermore there was no particular need for him to be in a state of deep relaxation. What was clear was that, I had simultaneously squeezed two nerve ends that likely caused the shock sensation. That was evidently the perfect catalyst causing the man to jump in reaction to a sharp pain. Whether it was the pain shock, the reactive little jump or the landing or all three combined - that combined reaction obviously made the important difference, which released the trapped nerve.

My conclusion is the man's innate healing intelligence understood and projected the precise support it needed, which I picked up telepathically to intuitively sense all that needed to be done. Therefore to me, saying I was the healer is like attributing a surgeon's scalpel as being the healer in an operation. This is obvious when it is clear only the patient's body or innate healing system can heal the wounds after the surgeon has done his work of cutting and sewing the parts together in the best way possible.

It was such experiences of something I can only describe as healing on the hoof that further caused me to reflect deeper into how the innate healing intelligence worked. Despite many hours of analysis, intuition and telepathy, undoubtedly they were to stand out as the foremost important factors. When one notable spontaneous healing occurred in front of my eyes while walking in a crowd of people, this alerted me to even greater healing possibilities. This was not perceived as a license to interfere in people's lives or their ailments willy-nilly but simply offer the ideal solution as and when situations presented themselves to me via the soup of energy and information. Those and other experiences were all part of an on going learning process. Such events confirmed that healing can be affected at almost any time or place, even in the hubbub of a crowded street, hotel swimming pool or even as in another occasion in a busy airport waiting lounge.

Consequently my intuitive notion was constantly pushing me to break down the boundaries of possibility and start thinking about the meaning and diversity of alternative support healing in a fundamentally different way. In the end it is all so simple. Since the real healer is inside the patient or sufferer all I have ever been needed for has been to cause a shift in subconscious changes, usually to permit the healing of traumatised emotions.

In the process of studying the writings of progressive doctors, surgeons and current medical and neuroscience research, I discovered another world of a general awareness of how the human body is supported by incredible survival and regenerative self-healing systems. The key to this organisation is a stunning intelligence and communication systems between every cell and every part of the body all bound together by a mind boggling DNA management program and not forgetting those vital centres of intelligence.

One of the most illuminating research papers to come to my notice concerned senescence programs. This opened up an entirely new study and eventual understanding of a little more about how the body manages itself. Even so the important question kept arising as to when it stops doing that, why and what has changed?

These research papers showed that highly skilled research teams were struggling to understand how specific parts of the body system work. Therefore, for me trying to understand everything about all the possibilities of how such intelligence could become blocked or switched off, was clearly trying to do what the most advanced research institutes around the world had not been able to do so far. Thus it was practically impossible for me to do the same or better. At the same time I had the intuitive insight why in any event that line of thinking was in my case completely unnecessary. All I had to do was to lean what were the essential issues and then seek the guidance of the patient's all knowing innate centres of intelligence. I had already taught myself how to activate intuitive intelligence on demand. Therefore, the key was to first give the assurance I had no intention of interfering but was only interested in supporting as appropriate. Then I could assist in spontaneously re-activating this incredible inner healing intelligence.

In view of my experience with certain exceptions, it is clear alternative healing therapy is essentially a complementary support filling in the missing link when orthodox medicine has no more answers. Most; probably as much as 95% of those people who came to me did so as a last resort when the doctors had no more solutions. It was therefore, somewhat ironical the day my childhood doctor came to me for healing. He was now in his nineties, greatly overweight and with a serious heart condition. Both his hip joints were badly eroded so walking was painful at best. At that time the hospital surgeons would not operate due to his age and the risk of a general anaesthetic on his heart. Every week he came for healing but no one was fooled. We both agreed the healing was aimed at easing his discomfort rather than persuading his innate healing system to build him two new hip joints, while also fixing his heart. The healing certainly did bring him relief for several days after each support healing session. It was also just as much an excuse to have a chat about his life and the growth of medicine, how my healing worked and generally put the world and politics to rights.

It showed me how word got around even though I tried to be discrete. I never said no to anyone, but my boyhood doctor asking me for support healing was slightly daunting. Bizarrely, working with someone with terminal cancer caused me no problems as on so many occasions it all turned out well. I did not keep a track of the months he came to see me, then one day he did not make his appointment. A few days later his wife called to say he had had another heart attack and was no longer with us. Although he realised his time was soon up, he died happy and what little I did for him certainly eased his persistent pains during those last months, so that was not so bad.

Mankind has relied on and been supported by many healing beliefs, placebos and superstitions for thousands of years, as such we have survived to tell the tale. In the middle ages our greatest health hazards were water so polluted that gin was mixed with it simply to sterilise it. Of course there were wars, the pox, lethal accidents, bad hygiene, poor food and rotting teeth. All in all it seems Neanderthal man had a better life some thousands of years earlier. Clean fresh stream water, no wars, only the odd tiger or bear to disturb their tranquillity. There is a mass of archaeological evidence indicating that primitive Neanderthal man actually had a budding health service. Approximately from 41,000 and 200,000 years ago, they were using caring skills including what we would refer to as surgery today. Archaeological evidence of Stone Age surgery such as trepanning also setting broken bones, suggests these operations were a common practice. Therefore, clearly there were specialists trained and experienced in this healing work. Undoubtedly intuition and telepathy must have played an important part in that evolutionary process. They must have learnt that bones will glue themselves together, so why not put them back in their former position and restrict movement until healed. The fact that so many bones have been found, which had been perfectly joined, gives credence to deductive, intuitive and telepathic skills enabling those early operations to be so successful.

Trepanning or the opening of holes through the top of the skull, are believed to have been for the purposes of releasing cranial pressure. Perhaps this was after falling rocks, a depressed skull with serious pain or disability, a big stick during a fight or perhaps due to a hunting injury. Possibly trepanning was carried out to relieve other forms of persistent head pain. Some speculation believes it was to release troublesome spirits. In one interview a specialist archaeologist concluded those who performed the trepanning and setting of bones had a considerable knowledge of human anatomy. In some instances more than one hole in the same scull had fully formed new protective bone. This is important as it indicates the person receiving the trepanning lived many years after their operations.

Over these enormous time spans it is inevitable that the Sharman or medicine man or woman evolved and then gradually gained a substantial knowledge of what worked and what to avoid. They were certainly relying on observation and very likely had developed their intuitive and telepathic awareness to a higher level than we are conscious of today. Only via the intelligence to test the ideas they sensed to be worthwhile, could they improve their methods, find new practices and so start the process we know today as medical science and neuroscience.

From North American Indian traditions it is known they developed a belief in the healing spirits of the earth, trees, wind, rain, water, sun, as well as a number of animals. Across the expanse of Asia, shamans or healers believed in the power of nature and balance of energy. These were the critical influences and forces affecting their lives. Consequently it is reasonable to conclude that is where they would have believed themselves to draw inspiration. They developed more than just healing skills. It is also evident how they began to understand the power of the conscious and the subconscious mind.

Eventually those learnt skills that were reliable developed into the healing arts of modern shamanism, spiritual healing and the study and practices of herbalism and then into the science of homeopathy. Part of the healing arts split off and became what we know today as the accepted establishment of the orthodox medical profession. Hippocrates in 460BC was the first accredited to have made logical sense of the body and disease. Two thousand years later circa, 1489, Leonardo da Vinci began his book "On the Human Figure" in order to really explain how the human body actually worked. His famous detailed drawings taken directly from dissected corpses depicted the inside workings of the human body and so medical science gradually evolved and accelerated over the following centuries into the modern orthodox medicine we recognise today.

Another spin-off of ancient pre-history was to become Chinese plant medicine, which required a great deal of experience and study. Acupuncture is also known to have taken a very long time to evolve. As the incredible complexity of acupuncture emerged, some believe about six thousand years ago, others record this as two thousand or fifteen hundred years BC. However some archaeologists consider that given the skills of trepanning, acupuncture may have evolved from and as far back as our cave man ancestors. Whatever, it is based on invisible energy meridians that could only have become known via intuition and observation. Today those meridians are detectable by extremely sensitive monitoring equipment proving those beliefs to be more natural science than mythic folk law.

A similar thing happened in India where the tradition of Ayurveda medicine, including a mixture of balancing energy flows, yoga, herbalism and other studied observations evolved to become a well tested form of both preventative and healing medicine. Because of their completeness and effectiveness, over the past several decades acupuncture and Ayurveda medicine have gained considerable attention and popularity in the west.

The key to Ayurveda and Chinese medicine healing is to treat all the parts, the mind, body and body/mind at the same time. I only became aware of some of the intricacies of Ayurveda and Chinese medicine when I was well into researching my own support healing. As my knowledge of all three developed I realised my own support healing was not simply a standalone healing. Because the patient was their own healer, their innate healing system performed at its best in conjunction with medical science also other therapies.

During my research into my own healing gift I have certainly understood the importance of negative also paradoxically positive traumas and the emotional energy involved within. Now when I talk about holistic therapies, I am conscious of the need to understand so much more about emotional intelligence. With its powers to dictate involuntary responses to the events that lead to emotional traumas; there is a great need to understand exactly what is involved. Just as much as there is a need to support the healing of the traumas themselves, there is a need to ensure we do not interfere in an intelligence we are only now barely scratching the surface of.

How careful must we all pay attention to Hippocrates and his advice; "whatever you do, be sure to do no harm."

THE PLACEBO FACTOR

The placebo effect is well known in orthodox medicine with doctors largely split evenly as to its dangers, its values, effectiveness or importance. The process is frequently used when doctors believe their patient is suffering from a psychosomatic (emotionally controlled) condition. Doctors know their patients have an expectation to be given pills or medicine and they will get better. This faith and belief in the doctor is in itself the basis of the placebo effect, while the sugar pills close the circle of expectations.

(*Psychosomatic conditions are as a rule triggered by stress about an emotional problem, which manifests itself as a physical condition. The placebo phenomenon exhibits an interaction between the psychological and the physiological by recognising and meeting beliefs, values and expectations.*)

I have often wondered if the placebo method of treatment is some doctor's way of respecting the rule of "whatever you do, be sure to do no harm." If the harmless sugar pill does the trick then the condition was psychosomatic. If the placebo did not work, no harm is done and the doctor then has a better idea of finding the problem and a better solution. Of course in the 21st century there is a blood test to identify practically any health condition, thus the guess work and trial by error should be largely superseded by laboratory analysis.

Despite the above diagnostic technology, the important yet simple act of sharing worries with a respected person like a doctor, alternative healer or someone you value, is known to have a considerable psychologically healing benefit. This can be a placebo in its own right.

I grant that this is essentially faith healing but that idea is a potential trap. Do not forget the length of training the doctor needs to understand a psychosomatic condition also that he or she is licensed to practice this level of "faith" healing. Pure faith healers neither have the training nor licensed to practice orthodox medicine. This is why in my own support healing the only healing intelligence I rely on is that of the patient's innate healing systems own impeccable intelligence to know exactly what the cause is and precisely the ideal support it needed from me.

Although convinced I was not the healer, patently part of the key to healing is being honest with myself as well as my patients. Only many years after beginning the healing process; was there a fuller understanding of the innate healing system and its intelligence. Then I was able to explain to my patients, why I believed they were their own greatest healer or their greatest stumbling block. This led to explaining exactly what I meant and how I believed not interfering was so important.

I found this honesty was important for me also I believe it was vital to the patient's innate healing intelligence. That is, it indicated how I respected and put the power and responsibility where it belonged. This certainly worked for pragmatic thinkers who were interested and somewhere relieved to discover my support healing was explainable. However, the faith issue does inevitably creep into the equation as many patients arrived by recommendation. This meant they already had confidence and therefore faith knowing their friends or acquaintances apparently had been healed by me.

This approach did not work for everyone as there were occasional patients who were strong believers in the spirits of divine healing. Because they believed orthodox medical doctors and their treatment had failed them they would have no truck with my explanations of how the body can heal itself given a fair chance. For spiritually devoted people having been through dashed hopes of often challenging treatments, my assertions though practical to me, could easily cause offense to others.

Diversity of people and our beliefs and values is what makes the world go around although we may not understand why. Tim Spector says in his book "Your Genes Unzipped."

"Genes can influence virtually all aspects of our lives, and as a consequence some readers may be depressed and others may be relieved. Yet there is still a significant role for conscious decision making in altering our behaviour and environment. Understanding this explains why humans are so diverse and unpredictable."

The above quote says a great deal about the importance of knowing ourselves and being fully conversant with what is important to us. Apart from everything else genes are responsible for; they also determine our intuitive and telepathic intelligence awareness. This is how we listen to our inner or subconscious intelligence. When we know ourselves at the subconscious level then we really are connecting to a far greater dimension of who we really are. Thus given this understanding, connecting to this intelligence changes how we access so much more of our largely uncharted potential.

I do accept this uncharted potential; can be for many an opening to realising their spiritual needs. I have spoken about the spark of life being incredibly fragile also having unbelievable resilience. I speak about scientists at the CERN research facility striving to find what has become known as the God factor or the origin of the spark of life. Ultimately it does not matter what the scientists find or what any of us choose to believe in. So long as it is out of love and therefore what does us the most good, then we can do no harm.

Controlled deep reflective meditation or trance enables us to momentarily let go of conscious and habitual automatic limiting thinking patterns and our deepest spiritual beliefs. The main question is if we can accept this subconscious wisdom. This is because it will inevitably challenge us to step out of the box, to think and even to believe in a different way.

There is another important issue in using this self awareness. It is to master the act of letting go. When making major decisions, we hope to make the best choices. So often we fall into the trap of repeating old preferences rather than rationally thinking what is really best. The main problem is that conscious reasoning has little idea of all the consequences available to us in making our choices. Whereas, given the principle that subconscious intelligence knows what the future is, subconscious intelligence does not have to explain the detail it just makes the right choices for us provided we have the confidence to access its intelligence and accept it as trustworthy.

Equally, as it is impossible to master all the workings of the brain and innate healing system so it is practically impossible to know and understand all the potential outcomes of any change action. The above suggests we subjugate ourselves to an intelligence we do not understand. It is essentially putting the cart before the horse. Put in the reverse order, we then understand this intelligence is part of us, therefore trusting in it is learning to trust our greater potential rather than some mysterious spiritual guidance. What may make this trusting difficult to accept is in part because we always had it but learnt to ignore it simply because we had never before learnt how to use it other than by default. Therefore why not use it to our greater advantage. After all it is all about better self leadership and greater use of what is at our service for perhaps a way of life beyond self delusion. This demonstrates that it is better to know ourselves fully. Understanding and believing in ourselves and the power of our subconscious intelligence, is far better than believing in dogmas invented by others for their own benefit, who may not have our own best interests at heart.

Thus, with practice and guidance, deep meditation combined helps to achieve access to the highest degree of subconscious high performance. Once high performing meditation techniques are adopted and mastered, they take all the time consuming focused concentration out of the meditation. One begins to understand the sense of this as we go beyond meditation as a means and end in itself. Then the meditation becomes a means to informing the powerful subconscious intelligence precisely what we want it to do for us automatically. This has to be the smart way of using our brains in the future as principally it avoids stress as our evolving world becomes so much more challenging.

Paradoxically, I realised this is what I encapsulate in the words "brutal honesty" as I worked my way forward out of burnout. I decided on the words "brutal honesty" as they stripped bare any frills of fictitious imagination and wishful thinking, thus it gives no quarter for anything but squeaky clean self knowing truth.

Growing up in the late 1940s and 1950s it was considered de-rigueur within the social circles of my parents to protect children from the truth and many realities of life. As a young boy, I rarely saw and barely knew or understood my father. After he died when I was eight years old, this resulted in me unknowingly falling victim to my own imagination of unsafe presumptions as I tried to know and model him. Years later reflecting on this start in life, I realised I had been modelling my perceptions on largely my self-created myth, not the real man. Only in my fifties was I to discover much of his absence and mystery was to do with his involvement with military matters during the II World War of a sensitive nature. This explained much but not all about not knowing much about him and thus part of the reason for being protected from the whole truth and realities of life and career. Thus, as I began to understand these facts, I found knowing and understanding the brutally honest truth had a specific meaning of consequential importance to my appreciation of why proportionally there were so many gaps in knowing myself.

A spin-off of this process developed into a significant intuitive awareness. For some time the moment I encountered missing information, misinformation or someone intent on deliberate deception, my intuitive bells begin chiming. This was all very nice but until I better understood how it worked, it could lead to frustrations and uncertainty. One case was when at school or on a training course, I could frequently see where the teacher or instructor was headed but felt vital information was seemingly missing. Whether that was deliberate or the course material had not been well structured, I had no idea but evasive answers to my questions did not improve the situation. Thus slow or limited dissemination of information had the frustrating feeling of deliberate secrecy and therefore a feeling of distrust. We all have this intuitive awareness intelligence of who we naturally trust even though we may not understand why.

Getting to know myself has lasted throughout my life. Gradually I discovered unknown facts about my parents and grandparents. This meant the more I understood about the thinking and beliefs of my near relatives albeit they were dead, the more I understood the reasons for my own beliefs and thinking patterns, thus, the more I understood myself. My personal brutal honesty mantra first illustrated how in ignorance of the facts, I had created my own emotional stumbling blocks. It also pointed the way to change so I could make my way forward a little easier. The difficulty with this drip, drip process was that I found myself stumbling over my perception of my own identity. Eventually I could see the bigger picture. That was when I got the answer to my self-imposed questions, "What have I done to be able to do this healing thing and Why Me?" I have no delusion there is a spiritual hand at work. As medical science is continuing to understand with genome reading is that it is all down to our parents and ancestors gene programming

Curious to understand how all that happened, I found how children are incredibly capable of coping with the realities of life. They need the truth and reliable guidance so they grow mentally strong, confident and capable of assessing all situations wisely. In my experience the worst thing any of us can have is a life made up of half truths, innuendoes and over protection. The consequence is inevitably many gaping holes in our map of reality, identity, purpose and worldliness. Bereft of the truth and missing important facts is where we begin creating fictitious elements of our thinking and beliefs. If the box of protectionist security is what we learn to trust and rely on, all our own fictitious and imaginative distorted infillings are going to lead us astray or sooner or later they let us down badly. The moment or day we are forced out of our safety zone, is a principle cause of more stressors and subsequent high stress levels, which subsequently lead to constant failings and frustrations in finding our true identity and purpose.

The rewards are in really understanding who we are, our strengths and weaknesses. The fact remains that most of the beliefs and emotional baggage we carry around with us may not be us. Look carefully and we see how protectionism and distortions by our ancestors and parents, becomes the seed bed for unnecessary emotional baggage and more stress. There seems to be a growing divide between who we believe we are and who we really are. Therefore, protectionism from the whole truth like living in an alternative reality; gets in the way or downright prevents us from reaching our natural harmony and thus our greater potential and consequently it all eventually turns into more and more stress.

From this I am of the mind that being an entrepreneur was attractive to me mainly because I got to create my own reality and make my own rules. Even so due to my start in life I still had a tough time with my purpose and identity.

A greater understanding of working with the subconscious mind pointed me to discovering and understanding how centres of intelligence such as "Survival and Self Protection Intelligence" may both help or hinder us. I concluded that if by error we use this intelligence in the worst way possible, we are at risk it becoming the guidance that locks us inside our own box and that restricts our development.

As the case of the chronic depressive demonstrates, in extreme cases, survival and self protection intelligence when dealing with prolonged chaos can shut down reliable beliefs, values and behaviours. These are the stepping stones that help us to move forward again. If we shutdown these pillars of survival thinking, we are at risk of turning survival into a way of life rather than using wisely in restoring abundance thinking.

The action or implicit centre of intelligence is unable to differentiate between good or bad, positive or negative. Implicit intelligence is designed to do exactly as it is told to do. This is how and why we develop both good and bad behaviours and habits; the implicit intelligence ensures those habits keep cycling around. This is why clear leadership in stepping back out of the box to take a look at the detail is so important in preventing these intelligence paradoxes from harming rather than helping. Without this reflective assessment and analysis of our behaviours we just keep on making the same old mistakes and there is never any learning or change until something important breaks.

7th Sense Survival and Self Protection intelligence has its purposes when we are hit by chaos and trauma; it provides a place for healing. The "want to but cannot syndrome" can be caused when this process becomes stuck if it begins cycling around on itself. Recognising this self protection intelligence and reversing the process is extremely useful helping stuck states to release themselves so the person can move forward again.

A classic example of this negatively motivated psychological and neurological self destruction is in the case of Jim the businessman. He spent over a year progressively destroying his own company believing he was doing the right things to save it. His negative survival intelligence intuitively drove him into everything he was consciously fighting to prevent. Two years after the fall of his company, at his own instigation, it took about six hours of coaching to expose a train of thinking so he could recognise what he had actually done to bring about the very outcome he believed he was fighting to prevent. Much the same process helped Thomas the chronic depressive to break out of his self induced deep cave reclusive mentality; created to protect him from losing joy, happiness and friends before he had even got them.

Earlier I discussed the unusual possibility of healing in any situation no matter how noisy or chaotic. Being in a state of hypnosis, deep meditation or ultra deep relaxation is certainly an ideal environment for any healing. But regarding this as a hard and fast requirement is clearly mistaken thinking. This overlooks many healing situations and possibilities I have encountered, for example in the cases of the bent old woman walking in a crowd of people or a man standing beside a busy hotel swimming pool. A family reeling at the loss of their rock and leader also the woman with lifelong untreatable stomach pains dominated by a belief system and chaperones neither of which wanted her to be relieved of her condition. These and many other experiences of healing indicate the degree of subconscious connection, i.e. intuition, telepathy and allowing ourselves to be shown what is possible in everyday situations and not being limited by unchallenged beliefs.

Of course if a patient's mind is turning nineteen to the dozen in fear of their medical condition or because of many other related consequences, then to some degree a deep hypnotic calming may be required, nonetheless this may be extremely difficult to achieve because of the internal mental chaos. There is a useful alternative, which bypasses the concept of deep relaxation. A diversionary distraction, so ably done with life coaching methods may interrupt a powerful internal panic that blocks everything including their own innate healing intelligence. A sufficiently evocative coaching question known as "provocative coaching" may sometimes break any negative or emotional log-jam or performance stumbling block. Once this is cleared the patient's innate healing intelligence can get on with the job. Provocative coaching may not always work with everyone. Because it is effectively interference, depending on its use, some people will be jolted out of their limiting self protection shield, others simply put up a mental barrier. In the case of the latter, the support healer then has a subconsciously hostile patient, which is almost certain to prevent the all important telepathic link from happening between patient and healer.

WHERE TO FOCUS ATTENTION

The case studies of the crippled racing car driver also two cancer sufferers, examines how their inner intelligence or subconscious body control systems prevented recovery via medical treatment. In these cases even surgery and powerful pain killers were blocked by the body from doing their job. However, at a prescribed time, the perfect healing treatment that only took minutes with no drugs or surgery proved all that modern medicine could not do. This does not say the medical profession is wrong. In these cases they simply missed the fact that every medical condition invariable has psychological and neurological connections of body and mind.

As I have already explained, it may help the healer therapist to be aware of the problem but it is not wise to know the root cause. Knowing the details may be a trap for the healer or coach in believing they know the perfect remedy. Provocative coaching is an example that can backfire thus amounting to unwarranted and unhelpful interference. My conclusion is that provocative coaching is interference because it is essentially a cop-out when a coach of any description is not sufficiently focused on the coachee's subconscious intelligence.

Herein also lies the issue that a healer is not a qualified medical doctor, therefore, in any event, from both a medical and legal perspective, they are advised not to cross that red line. If an alternative healer wants to cross that line, as far as I am concerned they are also crossing psychological lines that speak of perceiving themselves to be the real healer. Not only is this a very slippery slope to interfering by thinking they know what is best for their patient they will automatically send the wrong telepathic message to the patient's innate healing intelligence and that will block any healing.

Traditional psychologists and psychotherapists are criticised for holding onto their patients far longer than necessary thus eventually causing a dependency. Maintaining an eye on a patient after healing, may to some extent be justified. When Jim the businessman who had destroyed his own twelve million pound company decided he had the answer he came for. No doubt due to his limited finances, this factor had an influence on him considering he was fixed and did not need the expense of more coaching or therapy. The result was he descended into, (in his own words) *"the bottom of a dark barrel."* It took him a year to emotionally climb out of this survival and protection barrel/cave and back to the confidence to think about his future in moving forward into a new business.

For the same reasons many modern surgeons specialising in facial cosmetic surgery, insist on the patient accepting psychological support before and after the operations. Thus also some healing needs backup support to make sure the patient does not embark upon the same psychological self fixing mess as Jim and others have done. This same process occurred in the case of the Spanish doctor. Before I saw him, he knew he only had two weeks or so before being taken into hospital for intensive care to ease his dying. Two weeks later he was not in hospital but in his surgery. Cured of the cancer he was miraculously doing what he loved the most, helping his patients. Like Jom the entrepreneur, even though he was an experienced doctor, his reprieve turned into a massive self induced, emotionally driven self-recriminating psychological catastrophe. The learning curve can indeed be exceedingly steep and troubling. The doctor had some special beliefs of his own about spiritual healers. I was pleased to hear of the doctors recover and never for a moment considered such a thing could happen in his case.

Just like this doctor, part of the months that followed Jim's coaching breakthrough were taken in psychologically reconciling his past thinking process that had created the problem in the first place. Neither businessman Jim nor the Spanish doctor contacted me to mention the emotional chaos or agony they were in. This is another example of why, when no matter what state or degree of trauma, one should avoid trying to go it alone. A support healer or life coach should also give just waning and keep an eye on patients or clients, especially when a dramatic change occurs quickly.

WHEN INNATE INTELLIGENCE DOES NOT KNOW

There are numerous cases of spontaneous remission to surprise doctors where people suddenly find they are free of any trace of their ailment. These bear witness to the mind body/mind's ability to heal itself perfectly and quickly once that inner intelligence and inner healer understand there is a problem and have decided the conditions are right for self healing.

Dr. Deepak Chopra MD, makes reference to the power of the innate healing intelligence in his book Quantum Healing. (Chopra Deepak, 1998) He says, *"The frustrating reality, as far as medical researchers are concerned, is that we already know that the living body is the best pharmacy ever devised."*

Okay, so what are the medical researcher's frustrations if the body is capable of such wondrous things? The answer is in not understanding why this amazing system does not work all the time, or stops working and can even work against itself or indeed work against otherwise reliable medicines.

This is the same scenario as to why one patient's responses to healing can be quite different from that of other patients with the same medical problem. The answer was in understanding how psychologically and emotionally the mind body/mind can shut down or block a natural healing process or appropriate medication if the innate healing intelligence does not recognise there is a problem. This clearly indicates that mind, body and emotions need to be considered in any medical intervention or alternative healing.

Have the big pharmaceutical companies lost the healing plot as the lure of massive profits and a captive clientele expand? Have the Big-pharmaceutical companies fallen into a trap of kill or cure? They continue to create ever stronger drugs of incredible complexity with the purposeful intention of smashing through the body's defences and its own innate healing intelligence systems to force their medication to do the healing. I see this as similar to provocative coaching, when subtlety does not work in cracking the nut then use a sledge hammer and their policy is the more powerful the better. The obvious problem with this approach is that many of those medications are very dangerous and like the sledge hammer approach invariably they do a great deal of collateral harm to the body's own survival, immune and healing systems. What on earth has happened to working with the body's innate intelligence and do no harm?

The Hippocratic Oath: (Modern Version) *"I swear to fulfil, to the best of my ability and judgment, this covenant: I will respect the hard-won scientific gains of those physicians in whose steps I walk, and gladly share such knowledge as is mine with those who are to follow."* This plays into the pharmaceutical companies and some doctors' hands and neatly bypasses Hippocrates' own advice.

LEARNING FROM OUR ENVIRONMENT

Discipline is the key. This discipline is intended as a way of life and for life. Stopping the discipline or only respecting it periodically is like no longer or only occasionally putting oil in your car's engine, its hydraulic steering or brake system when their reservoirs have dried up. Too little, too late makes for greater damage or suffering and more difficult and costly repairs. For us it is exactly the same. When our immune systems security reserves are depleted, we might breakdown with colds, flu or possibly with lumbago or sciatica or such conditions, which appear more frequently as a warning we are not listening to our own inner intelligence guidance.

When conditions develop that are more serious and require more than self medication via the local pharmacy, we clearly need the support and guidance of doctors and other medical specialists. Some people may prefer to live in blind faith of the orthodox medical system and not ask awkward questions. Questions like; how have I contributed to my conditions and what can I do to prevent this and other ailments happening again in the future.

Paul G. Thomas developed the science of Psycho-cybernetics in keeping ourselves on track by virtue of recognising when we are beginning to veer off-track. This may be easier to follow from the aspect of our daily, life or career goals. Mostly we put care of the cart of performance before the care of the essential horse, which is the motive power of performance. From a psycho-cybernetics point of view and remember this is our inner direction finder; if the horse that drives the cart of performance cannot see the road because the load of performance has been given greater importance and thus has become so enormous, then evidently sooner rather than later the whole thing ends up in the proverbial ditch.

Yes; we do have incredible innate body management and healing systems. The downside is we also have the willpower and foolery to override them. A very public example of this was when Hilary Clinton collapsed due to pneumonia in September 2016 during her presidential race to the USA White House oval office. During a telephone interview with a CNN news reporter, she admitted that she knew she was ill but said nothing and tried to power through. She said it was a one-off important occasion that she attended so she may be forgiven for making the effort. Regardless of this point of view that was the straw that broke the camel's back. It is not the one-off that does so much damage but the general accumulation of disregard for constant surveillance and care, which invariably brings us to a breaking point. Then all it takes is one more straw of irresponsibility to bring the whole system crashing to its knees.

As Clinton demonstrated, when under pressure, especially when we have specific motivations, we have the tendency to allowing self-determination to push ourselves to keep going despite the discomfort and risks. These behaviours usually are not isolated. Frequently they are established patterns of behaviour or habits. In Clinton's case, taking risks with her health have been recorded to be one of her repeated bad habits.

This is equivalent to putting a massive paper clip in place of traditional filament style electrical household fuses. Normally this is a fine hair like wire designed to fail only as a warning when under abnormal load. Paper clips and even nails have been found in place of purpose made electrical fuses. Many of those unfortunate security override adaptations have been responsible for burning houses and factories to the ground. Wilfully ignoring life's warning fuses of stressors, stresses, strains, bruises and overwhelming pressures, bolstering ourselves with personal pep talks, soldiering on and powering through when we know we are suffering, is when we are at greater risk of breaking down. Please note I write these words of dire warning through personal and bitter experience of the consequences of fully fledged burnout.

Why do grown intelligent people do that? There can be many unique reasons, however the main cause is because first, we allow stressors and stresses to occur and build up. We do this due to our thinking and performance patterns and strategies being out of harmony or synchronisation with who we are. We push our chosen purpose and ever greater demands for performance without understanding the appropriate mind sets necessary to do that successfully without stress. We also do this inadvertently by a bizarre perversion of willingly going through life blindfolded and laced with addiction to be seen to be superhuman. Every second, minute, hour and day of our lives we use and abuse the vehicle, which carries all the processes that sustain the spark of life. Little wonder we have such a massive health services industry.

In this case it is more self recrimination than lecturing because I recognised that is how I created my own burnout. As far as I see, the problem is we all need much more lecturing in order to give us better inner leadership and most importantly understanding why we are doing that. My burnout happened because like so many managers and entrepreneurs; I did not know and therefore did not understand the hidden risks, I did not even know there were risks of being addicted to my work. It is with this same mentality that we push ourselves to the precipice of both physical and mental ill health by virtue of what we are doing that we do not know the results of.

Companies may diligently observe health and safety regulations but there are no such rules for managing people and so it is common to push managers and their teams' for ever higher performance and results. My case was self imposed, I liked my work and I was good at it. I could not have imagined it was driven by addiction and this was a trap in itself. In both cases the end result is the same sustained high stress, which leads to life style imbalance, which leads to emotional and physical health imbalance. These are the frictions that cause excessive wear and tear and eventual breakdown or poor performance both of which are major stressors. Like stressed managers and entrepreneurs, or for example people with high debt, other seemingly insurmountable personal problems or chasing challenging goals to extremes, instead of leading myself from the front by being aware of all the pitfalls, I was ignoring myself in favour of and in most cases pushing my overloaded cart of purpose from behind so I was blinded as to where I was headed.

The other side of the burnout coin are people who settle with or into disharmony. This could be because they accept and put up with a life or job they dislike or hate. That can be due to being in the wrong job or inadequately trained for that position. That is why we are constantly fighting an internal forest fire of catch-up, self doubt, fear of the whole thing collapsing and panic. The irony is we are all responsible for creating the fire for ourselves. As a businessman I lit multiple forest fires of renewed stress by jumping at contracts that were a real challenge. This fired up all my creative imagination that I knew kept my companies in the vanguard of the competition. That also fired up the production of more adrenalin and so I fed my addiction to overwork. What I regarded as performance had become counter-performance because I was effectively driving an express train that was out of control. In hindsight it is now clear that it would either jump its tracks or crash headlong into the buffers.

There may be many good examples of a better way. One I came to be familiar with as part of my work was that of British layers, solicitors and barristers. In reflection I realise how they deal with highly stressful situation while not subjecting themselves to the stress. In a few words they remain highly focused but detached. They do what I had done with my support healing in never taking my patients' troubles on my own shoulders. This seems to be an alternative method to achieving high performance without high stress.

In the world of coaching there is an exercise called the wheel of life. It consists of a pie chart and each segment represents an important part of life. These segments can be adjusted to meet all needs. They include work, play, sports, study, family, friends, relaxation, enjoyment, love and so forth. Each segment is not just about how large or small they are. The quality and degree of effort, interest or intensity are the factors that change the depth of each segment. The finished wheel indicates how balanced or usually unbalanced our lives really are. This is patently visible in the fact there is no one smooth exterior circumference to the wheel. Invariably it is rough, castellated and far from smooth running. The final stage of the exercise is to imagine putting that wheel of your life on your car or a bicycle and just what kind of bumpy uncomfortable ride your life style is actually giving you?

When we are under the control of copious quantities of the hormones cortisol and adrenalin they change the way we think.

normal rational thinking goes out of the window to be replaced with something else. As a rule that might be constant irrational quick fixes and knee jerk reactions that are meant to smooth out the road but invariably make our situation and journey worse. In this state when we should be focusing on the process and the finish line we are mainly focused on our discomfort and emotional turmoil. That has the spin-off consequence of also focusing on all the negative aspects of everything in our lives. Because stressors are bonded firmly to emotional energy and its intelligence, when we concentrate our emotional intelligence on our stressors we add more energy to those unhappy issues. The accumulation of all the above spontaneously drives the whole process of steadily rising internal stress.

What do most people do in this situation? They use the paperclip/nail, Hilary Clinton power through self-speak option of, *"I cannot be seen to be incapable, weak or ill, I will push on, try to overcome the problem with whatever resources are temporarily close to hand and maybe the subsequent problems will sort themselves out; by the way will ya pass that bottle of whisky and a paper clip."*

Successful ironman contestants train their minds and work with their coaches on improving mind strategies as much as they train their body. Every day normal life is becoming like an ironman contest but where is the team of performance coaches to support us? Where is the training to help us with the level of planning and preparation we all need just to go about our lives trying to do our best? Where is the guidance to help us understand the change in thinking behaviours needed to support a modern life? Where is the guidance to help us to fully understand and adapt to a life that has changed from challenging but comprehensible to a permanent competitive race. Where is; what should be the first line defence of our lifetime plan. Where is the training and education to wake us up to the importance of who we are, how the world of achievement works and the importance of knowing ourselves? Where are the values, guidance and understanding of what we need to do for ourselves in order that we can achieve high performance without high stress and finally messing up our lives?

Without this support in how to stay the course, rise to our own and other people's expectations, keep our jobs, our homes, families, mortgages, car, etc, all we do is build stress. My attention to myself after burnout taught me all those things and many more. In the most brutal manner this new view of my life woke me up to understand life is consistently this challenging and the more past mistakes the greater the challenge. Without breaks for resourcing ourselves, seriously analysing where we are, where we are going, how far we have got, what state of fitness are we in, what we need to sustain us during the continuing journey and how we will fill those needs, we face a life of more struggle than reward and that is just to stay in the game. If this is the case we have not the slightest understanding of what lies ahead or how to handle the good times let alone the bad. In a forward rush of mostly ill-conceived decisions, we so easily find ourselves making constant U-turns rather than consistently moving towards planned goals. The consequential internal stress being set in motion out of sight and out of conscious awareness is important to how long we survive and how much joy we get out of life.

Caring for ourselves is not being wrapped in cotton wool and protected from the big bad world outside by endless security shields, which simply creates stressful distortions. As mentioned in an earlier chapter, I learn this due to be protected from reality as a young child. In principle we get out of life what we put into it. Caring for ourselves goes far beyond the more material things important in our lives. Caring is equally about ensuring we sustain the journey in the most comfortable and enjoyable way. It is about doing ourselves no harm to our health, self awareness, confidence, capability, sense of purpose, performance and therefore achieving the most fulfilling and nurturing life style while still stretching ourselves.

Modern machines and their engines, have failsafe artificial intelligence systems to shut them down if critical issues are failing. When those safety or survival mechanisms are activated, the engines stop and cannot be restarted until the causes are corrected. Those security systems are designed to stop us humans doing a lot of harm without first correcting the issues. Those systems are as failsafe in themselves as reasonably possible because we humans have a very bad habit of interfering and thinking we know what we are doing when really we are doing so much harm.

We humans have the same processes as I have written about already in the form of "Survival and self protection intelligence." Our problem is we also have the willpower to override its warnings. So often our preference is to push ourselves onward through the pain barrier, through mental tiredness, deep body fatigue and anything else we happen to trip over that is doing its best to slow us down for a very good reason. This is how and why burnout happens in a multitude of different ways and forms.

Burnout is the ultimate off switch that not even the most determined can power through. Believe me; I did my best and all that did was to activate an even more impossible hurdle, it is just not worth the damage it causes.

Driverless vehicles are a hot topic and certain to be our safer future once the boffins get the detail sorted out. When that is done we humans will be so much safer. It is not that we will not be able to interfere, do not worry we will always find a way to interfere. After so many centuries; interfering has become our second nature. It is deeply engrained, indelibly stencilled in our genes. Will we simply and finally get the message it is easier to let the system take the stresses and strain. Breaking the rules of the road, jumping the traffic lights, breaking the speed limits, make mistakes and causing general chaos and mayhem, even killing people, will it really be in the past? If we do finally achieve this utopia, our first and enduring problem or stressor, will be in overcoming the stresses of no option but to let go and let the autonomous car intelligence drive with perfection.

Burnout for any that have experienced it and those who will inevitably come to know it, is a stark reminder that for some months before the burnout crisis, and for possibly four years after, the victim no longer has full reign of their life. You think that is bad, bizarrely I have concluded it is at least one positive in a sea of paradoxical hardships. The willpower to override the body's survival and self protection intelligence is in one stroke - shut down - no through way.

Full blown burnout is like being driven by an autonomous car. There is no more freewill to interfere or muck-up again even to do much else for that matter. We become like those high-tech machines with their artificial intelligent fail safe systems. No more is there a possibility of interfering and attempting to jump the traffic lights of our lives. As far as I can be certain it is principally our 7th sense survival and self protection intelligence supported by the implicit brain intelligence and subconscious ambition, who are in control.

Information on any of these or other principle centres of intelligence may be obtained at www.neurofaultprotection.com

This unleashed "change thinking control mechanism" blocks any capability to do anything remotely associated with what we did before to cause the burnout. Because for the time being we have no option but to slow down to a snail's pace, I observed that decisions slow down too. This is concluded to be because the "want to but cannot syndrome" blocks practically anything that is not thought through carefully. A new wisdom appears to show itself and that is when one begins to be aware of taking on an unfamiliar measured attitude to all aspects of life.

The intelligence of this syndrome has some sophisticated strategies to show us exactly how our lives should be managed. First it allows us to think and plan precisely what we are going to do to get back into harness. Next it allows us to actually begin putting our plans into operation complete with the necessary investment and resources. Then with no warning this intelligence slams the doors of capability in our faces and again we become aware of this iron fist of protection. Despite warnings not to repeat mistakes, it is common to repeat this behaviour several times before waking up to the fact we are going nowhere fast other than wasting time and valuable resources.

In this situation I learnt there was no recovery, no going back to what I did before. There can never be any recovery because recovery is going back to what caused the burnout and that once activated is what the "want to but cannot syndrome intelligence" and the "7th Sense of Survival and Self Protection intelligence" is programmed to prevent. These two centres of intelligence are powerful in their own right. Then they are even more powerful because they are closely linked. Finally they are inextricably connected to emotional intelligence, perhaps the most powerful of all internal management intelligence programs. Combined they are a perfect example of the sum total being far greater than the individual parts. Believe me, there is no escape. I tested them all to the limit with the relentless drive of a maverick workaholic.

The only possibility was to stand still. Moving forward at most crept into action after the healing and the realisation and understanding what had happened. Then came the acceptance of why it had happened and that the only way was forward into something totally different and even then with my Inner Master's self protection hand firmly on the tiller of my future.

Fail to observe this life stands still again until the penny drops. The hard won lesson is we may only move forward by letting go of trying to be in control especially when we are not fully aware of unseen consequences. Invariably there is a lot of emotional healing to be done. This may well be supported by life coaching as the main aim is to undertake a considerable amount of constructive honest introspection without paradoxically beating oneself up.

The purpose of this self-analysis, soul-searching, heart-searching and anything else searching, is to help us to understand and accept where we went so wrong to be able to throw such a massive spanner in the midst of our lives. It is the advice of Henry Ford when he said, "find what went wrong, what were the contributory mistakes and be sure never to do any of that again."

You will by now have likely realised that the use of this so very real burnout experience has become a synonym for all the bad things we do to ourselves during our lives. Medical scientists now understand that aging is the number one illness with the greatest mortality rate before our potential life span has run its course. Aging corresponds to the amount of damage we do to our brain, body, mind and all the component parts.

The subtlety of the 7th Sense Survival Intelligence is in that self-analysis process. Here we are strongly advised to drop any masks and even some serious limiting beliefs in order to begin to discover and eventually accept who we have become as a result of burnout. The next step is accepting life will never be as it was before. Therefore it is just as well we begin learning how to be closely observant of the one or if we are extremely lucky, one or two success behaviours or skills that had underpinned all previous successes. Doing this on one's own does take time and that is provided one is familiar with life coaching methods. Seeking the support of a life coach will almost certainly accelerate this process and avoid so many pitfalls and thus perhaps speed-up the overall healing process. To prevent the option of burnout go for the pre-emptive option of self respect, love and care for self and others and life balance.

There is one vitally important issue to understand about stress and stressors. No one and no thing or event purposely causes us stress. It is the emotional values we attach to people, things, places or events that trigger emotional stressors within our own feelings. A stressor can be seeing or hearing a person we cannot tolerate. We cannot tolerate them because their behaviours and beliefs clash with our own values.

A stressor can be a task like the case of many young managers being faced with having to address public speaking or giving a vital company presentation to someone important or to the board of directors. For a week in advance and a week after, they can be in perpetual panic. A stressor can be someone in the background that has no idea of the effect their behaviour is having on someone else's feelings and emotions. Stress is our internal friction when we cannot rationalise our beliefs, values, and responsibilities with the surrounding environment and the people in it.

There are two principle solutions to any such circumstances. First is to change our beliefs, values and behaviours to suit the stressful circumstances. In short, "When in Rome do as the Romans do." If there is no rub there is no friction and therefore there is no stress. If this is not an agreeable option or it fails for other reasons, then the solution is to quietly remove ourselves from the stressful situation. As this may not be practical there is a more powerful solution of programming the subconscious mind to intercept the stressor before it does its damage.

We create stress in ourselves when we choose to accept something that conflicts with our beliefs, balance and harmony without taking action to change or stop it. Distorted priorities, over-demanding performance relative to skill levels or endlessly being pushed, pushing or rushing to meet deadlines become our stressors, which directly impact negatively on emotional intelligence. Stressors are symptoms of performance expectations exceeding beliefs about capability and that can only end in more unnecessary stress.

Our stressors are all the irritating things we know are there also that we accept we have ignored or purposefully chosen not to confront. They are our missed opportunities and deep regrets. In many cases we are fearful to confront or change those issues because we do not know how to do that to the best effect. Alternatively, because of the presumed worst fall-out or backfiring scenario or other perceived or feared, seen or unseen consequences, we do little to help ourselves.

The longer we live with these stressors the more power they have over us and our emotions so once again they become the tail that wags the dog of stress also the cause of internal and emotional damage all of, which leads to faster aging. The cases of the elderly woman with lifelong stomach pains and "Quarry Workers" are perfect examples of this stress syndrome. When we reach this level we go through the motions of our own leadership but in truth we and our cause are already lost. Doing this too often or as a way of avoiding responsibility depletes self confidence. This shows itself in various ways so that other people see others as having no depth, substance or leadership. That is what so frequently causes certain capable employees to be overlooked for promotion or for the top job.

ANCESTORS AND EMOTIONAL BALANCE

Another problem arises when we are unaware that genetic behaviour patterns are being triggered by ancestral family alliances. Whether aware of these unusual behaviour patterns or not, a common automatic reaction can be that of some embarrassment, withdrawal,(freezing) forced laughter, (a form of running away) or instant aggression (fighting physically or by forcibly asserting one's ego image, which is a sign of protecting a vulnerability and a lie). These behaviours signal our stress levels are rocketing skywards and we have little or no idea of why we get into those situations. The best we can do is to recognise and note these specific patterns of behaviour. Unless one has analysis skills it may be best to consult a life coach who should be trained in how to guide us in finding the origins of those stressors or certainly preventing them from occurring spontaneously when not necessary.

Achievement, especially of the almost impossible, so often has a great deal to do with perception and the focal point of detailed observation. Changing the view point of perception will invariably change the outcome. This is related to seeing a cup half full or half empty. So, 'what if' we turn the cause and effect around?

Saying, *"I am constantly ill because I am powerless in my life and my immune system is weak,"* may be true but can be viewed as putting the cart before the horse. Thus it puts all the blame on the acceptance of an almost impossible situation instead of where the responsibility really belongs.

What if we say; *"my immune system is weak because I do little if anything to manage my situation, or care for myself and my health, consequently I am always ill."*

The first example is the victim attitude that has nowhere to go because it is phrased as a fact, thus it is perceived as impossible to change and therefore there is no incentive to change. The second example is recognition that if making some changes and doing something positive then the health will improve. Now the door is open for positive change.

Stuck in seeing the system is at fault and being the problem. This keeps us in the problem mindset always attuned to or focused on the problem. Accepting the immune system is weak because of what we are not doing, points our thinking towards the solution. Because we are in a solutions mindset, sooner or later the solution becomes apparent.

As we head into our fifties and older, our modern world of technology and ever growing "Big brother," social control and yes autonomous cars, becomes a growing source of stress. It becomes a stressor because a typical reactive behaviour is to run and hide from anything we do not understand or believe we cannot understand because it threatens our habits and way of thinking.

Interestingly, partial and then fully autonomous cars are something of an anomaly to our human condition. The development of the modern motor car is testament to our fascination with this form of transport. Fully autonomous electric cars will happen because global warming politics is certain to determine not if but when this will happen. Our lust for freedom and ease of travelling keeps us firmly wedded to the car. However, fully autonomous electric cars will possibly be the biggest worldwide mass emotional shock. As far as cars are concerned we are control freaks. This will be the biggest manifestation of the Big Brother syndrome. Over one hundred years of programmed expectations to do as we please behind the steering wheel of a car are going to disappear in one or two decades in first world countries. We might have to conform but stress levels will rocket as a result of this enforced change. Undoubtedly a new leisure activity will emerge. Like going to the gym, we will go to manual petrol or electric car driving arenas, complete with traffic lights, speed limits to ignore; in order to reduce our stress. Otherwise holidays in foreign countries still tied to their internal combustion non-autonomous cars offers the opportunity of hiring and driving old fashioned cars and breaking all the rules of the road with impunity.

A further stressor raises its horny head as we pass retirement age. Just as we automatically let go of so much we needed to stay in the game, we suddenly understand our lives still depend on being conversant with so many aspects of this modern world and its technological ways. We may not be able to change this but we are almost obliged to make the effort to stay abreast of the technology. The upside to this issue is that in learning these skills, we build confidence in our ability to compete at least at a reasonable level. Therefore, we wake up to the fact that life leaves us behind if we chose to opt out and opting out is a bad option. This is because it raises our stress levels and has the potential to push the less resilient into opting out of living before their natural time.

When examining your life closely from thirtyish onwards, the internal conversation might go something like this.

"I am feeling tired and have not been very well for some time. I sense I am under emotional pressure so I am being easy on myself by eating quick meals even so I am always in a rush. I know it is not that good but as I have so much to do, it gives me more time to work. However, I have the feeling I'm working harder and getting less done. Yes, I have been working too long hours or too hard for too long. In addition I have not been getting enough sleep because I know I am unhappy with my situation but I feel powerless and too tired to find any solutions and then when I do get some sleep I wake up feeling exhausted. I have not been getting enough relaxation or pleasure. I don't seem to have the time and frankly I'm not interested in holidays or sport anymore. I have been ignoring that feeling of rejection or being undervalued at work. Now I think about it, it has begun to really trouble me also I notice how my feelings at work are like a mechanical process. Before I enjoyed my work, I enjoyed my holidays and my sport. Now I get stressed just thinking about going to work. I have put off the application for a more responsible job, which I know I

should do but I am fearful of more rejection. I know I can do the job but others will probably think I am not adequately qualified. Oh well I better stay where I am and hope something comes along and things naturally change for the better."

This is no make-believe story. I have heard it said in one form or another on several occasions. Perhaps you too have had the same or similar thoughts during moments of reflection, and doubt about yourself and uncertainty of the future. This conversation tells a great deal about mounting stress, the depressing effects of limiting beliefs, false perceptions, missed opportunities, unrealised goals, awareness of outdated values, non-supportive environments and not knowing how to change things.

When reversing the process the internal conversation might go something like the following:

"I am aware of stagnating in my job and my life at a time when I should be heading to my very best. I saw that job advertised, which I am certain fits my skills and experience, what is more I feel I would enjoy the position and the challenge also the higher salary will enable me to take a more active life. What is more, there is a social side to the job, which means I will have more incentive to balance my life. I shall send my application today and see what happens. After all I have nothing to lose but my bosses will see I still want to develop my career and if they do not do something about it they may lose me to another company. Certainly I am aware of feeling undervalued at work, which probably means I have outgrown my position so if I do not get the job that shows it really is time for me to move on. My recent tendency to eating junk food quickly to give me more time to work is actually a false strategy. Believing that I have to constantly help other people unable to do their work properly is undermining my own results. Changing my job will mean a change of office location so that will break the habit of being the office helper and fixer. Yes, it is time I move my butt and apply for that new job."

We may not recognise the fact that depleted self confidence may occur because all that stress cortisol changes the way we think, primarily destroying self confidence, distracting our focus and draining our energy. These three consequences of sustained underlying stress prevent us from stretching ourselves with new and greater challenges. Part of that stress may be because we are not getting the recognition returns and positive feedback, which normally drives new motivation.

Chapter 18

SPIRITUAL CONNECTION

Some patients like the Spanish doctor, were clear about what was wrong with them and stoically accepted the inevitable. Perhaps beneath the tough exterior mask, they had not given up after all. I found people like this doctor were really still fighting, but usually amongst an incomprehensible mountain of confused stress laden ideas.

I refer to the often repeated thoughts and words "Why?" and "Why me?" or "What have I done to deserve this?" In general terms these questions are unanswerable other than by deep psychological understanding, DNA and personal life experiences and performance analysis. Even then, at best any answers are likely to be anecdotal and fragmented. Therefore, in any event these questions result in additional internal confusion and more emotional turmoil. Thus, the more the stress and turmoil, the less the innate healing intelligence is able to do its job.

Cancer for anyone must be a terrible emotional shock whatever juncture it comes in their life. For the Spanish doctor who brought healing to so many for so long, the injustice of cancer must have been more emotionally challenging even despite some advanced level of experience and understanding. In those days switched off senescence programs and the possibility to switch them on again in order to reactivate apoptosis or normal programmed cell death was in its infancy. This was not something an average general practitioner worried about too much, largely because it was just a new theory and that meant any viable solutions would be decades away.

There is no normality after facing permanent pain or death to find again your spark of life burning with a far brighter promise of a revived future. To be restored to good health from death's door step is understandably a joy. However, it is at risk of becoming a new significant trauma. This new trauma is the difficulty to accept and believe it will last. Without having been there it is impossible for the rest of us to understand what effect it has. How do cancer victims internalise the first trauma of discovering a cancer tumour. Wondering why them, what did they do to deserve this? Eventually after going through the additional traumas of treatment, the helter-skelter of raised and then dashed hopes comes the certain trauma of one's abnormal death. Then add the miracle of being healed by unknown forces and then once again but the reverse trauma of "will it last" - "why them?" "Why should they be one of the few people to be saved?" "What have they done to deserve this," it all takes on a somewhat reverse nonetheless challenging meaning.

Many may turn to spiritual beliefs as the way they can manage what is in effect their deliverance and in some senses a powerful emotional event. If a doctor or surgeon saves our life, we likely consider that wonderful, acceptable and understandable. When a healer without any medical training or surgical intervention does what the medical profession fails to do, then confusion reigns and reasoning returns to default. Having little or no idea how capable the body is at healing itself, given no wrong interference, illogically the recovery of one's health and life is put down to spiritual intervention.

Never mind being told about the medical and neurological reasons about the innate healing systems intelligence, albeit, they are mostly circumstantial and anecdotal, all that suddenly fades into the background as a confused logic points the finger at the only feasible but illogical answer of spiritual intervention.

Why spiritual intervention is so acceptable as a default is that by reason of it being an unanswerable question it satisfies no further need for additional enquiry. By definition of spirituality, we do not enquire into the mechanics of how spiritual intervention or be it God can heal a cancer tumour. In this thinking bubble, hardened realists having survived cancer in this manner, default to God's will is God's will and the subject stops there. Part of the default process is that we are taught to accept miracles as divine or supernatural. Do not ask questions especially when it is a gift. This may be completely irrational but that is how our minds have been programmed for thousands of years since the first concept of spiritual entities was invented. I hear so many people speaking of their spiritual needs and beliefs, I wonder if the concept is not increasing. This is not because people are returning to their churches and temples and seeking the word of God. It is more to do with stress, confusing, anomalies, uncertainty, fears and it is the idea it is all too complicated to unravel, which turns our daily world upside down in a trice.

One group of patients were those who had come to terms with themselves and the world and had apparently found peace in their impending death. There was no longer any fight left in them. I felt these people had switched off their spark of life themselves and thus to some extent also their inner healer. Therefore, it was difficult to find open lines of telepathic communication necessary to support them. Despite this challenge there were still the successes. Seeing this so often, I wondered if finding internal peace is all it is cracked up to be or indeed really the worst thing anyone can do. Therefore perhaps it is true that a little but not too much stress is actually good for us as it moves us to think how to change what we have that does not please us. If we think and dream we are still alive and we still have a spark of life to nurture.

The opposite group were those who fought so hard to live against all odds. This could be so strong they not only managed to block any access to their innate healer intelligence, they were actually blocking it from the remotest chance to be helped. They had perfected the art of interfering, par excellence!

When I said, I realised as a support healer I was the last chance saloon, these people proved this in immaculate detail. They could usually real off by heart, chapter and verse of every conceivable alternative therapy imaginable and what is more, they had tried them all. In one case of a cancer victim in Oslo, she had consulted three separate homeopathic cancer specialists without declaring any of them to the other two. When I arrived in her house I found a table dedicated to a triple pharmaceutical nightmare. Combined she was taking over seventy prescribed medications each morning. As a large part of this improvised panic strategy she apparently risked organ failure. Not content with the doctors she added a few extras of her own from local pharmacies. I suspected that was what was causing most of her weakness, dizziness and constant vomiting. This was confirmed by a visiting nurse as excessive on their own but potentially lethal when combined. Fortunately for her, her body rejected most of them, which likely saved her life in the short term. Once this was corrected the vomiting stopped and she felt much better in herself.

I found it somewhat alarming the visiting nurse knew about all this but had said nothing. Also I was dumbfounded that on raising the subject she was reluctant to contact the three specialists concerned. She said her professional code of ethics and the law did not permit her to interfere. Eventually she did when I pointed out the poor woman would likely succeed in poisoning herself long before she could possibly die of cancer.

Another difficult group to work with were those with a profound religious belief. Their main intention seemed to be to argue the power of their belief for the sole purpose of proving I could do nothing against the will of their God. As far as they were concerned, if I was instrumental in healing them it was God's will and if it did not work that was also God's will.

When they came to me for healing a cancer when the doctors had failed, their faith energy seemed to me to be the very disruptive interfering force that blocked healing from happening. I failed to understand fully why these people asked for my help in the first place. Why couldn't their God do the healing and cut out the competition. However each encounter was a lesson in how equally powerful the mind is to embrace pain, punishing spiritual beliefs and death as it is to accept the challenge of life, living, joy and happiness.

Many who came were at peace with their faith and their God. They had no need to impose their spiritual beliefs on me other than mentioning they prayed to God for his help. This group seemed to be fairly pragmatic about the fact that their God or their faith was not going to heal them. At the time I found it strange that with no limiting belief or obstacles, their healings were frequently quite satisfactory and unremarkable by the standards that had become a normal pattern.

LIMITING BELIEFS AND FEARS TURN US INTO VICTIMS

Earlier I mentioned one patient with constant stomach pains. This is a reminder of how religion, spirituality, fear and practicalities of life combined can play a controlling part in so many lives. Such emotions are a dark reminder of the terrible things done in the name of

God, both in the past and the present, across the world by those with strong unbending or radical beliefs.

The woman I have referred to arrived with two heavy set female guardians, appearing like a pair of Rottweiler guard dogs. The three sat side by side on a settee made for two, thus, making a bizarre spectacle. Those brooding dark guardian angels watched and carefully scrutinised every word spoken.

My patient explained she had endured terrible stomach pains for most of her life. Her doctors had never been able to find the cause or a remedy. Some years earlier she had joined a spiritual church and the church healers had no success so they concluded her pains were God's will. However she had heard about my healing and hoped I could help. The fact was fairly obvious that if I succeeded they and their church members were going to appear foolish if not incompetent.

I sat on a dinning chair in front of my patient with the chair-back between us; this was only to pacify these fearsome chaperones. Next I asked her coaching questions, which she calmly answered in full. After a few minutes of questions and answers, my patient began smiling.

"The pains have gone," she said.

Her guardian dogs of war looked across to each other with alarm. It was clear they were about as happy as if they were on a sinking ship in an ocean of confusion.

"It is amazing to be sitting here for the first time in my memory to be free of the pain," she said.

"In that case there is nothing else to be done. You may leave but come and see me next week so that I can verify all is well."

She and her troubled chaperones got up and left without a further word. Several days later the woman called me on the telephone to say she would not be coming back to see me again. She explained that when she went to her church on the following Sunday, she was happy to show all her friends and the minister that she was finally healed and free of pain.

She was shocked to find her chaperones had done their dark work well. Instead of rejoicing for her, she was roundly chastised by all the congregation for working with the devil to take away a pain that God had intended for her to suffer in repentance for all her sins.

As such she was sent from the church in disgrace. She then hesitated. *"All my friends are church members and none will talk to me. I cannot live alone; the church has been my life for so long, so I went to see the minister. He advised me to seek the forgiveness of God and take back the pain. He prayed with me and I prayed hard that the pains would come back. The next day I had the same pains again. The minister then blessed me and took me back into the church. I am sorry,"* she said and hung up her phone.

As sad as I find this story, it confirms my conclusion that in the first instance of our meeting, she had faced her emotional blockage. Despite her fearsome spiritualist church guardians, this woman let go of a fear and the dogma of her fellow church goers and then she was able to heal herself. All I did was to guide her by coaching to the point she accepted she had hidden from all her life. In those moments she had understood something important about herself and the reason for hanging onto the pains.

I remember during the coaching how her facial expressions changed rapidly. These were apparently indications a great deal of processing was going on in her brain. Finally she sorted out whatever was stuck. She confessed to knowing what she had been hiding from all along but did not realise it could cause her such pains. The next facial change was her smile like a child opening the most fabulous Christmas present.

It was clear to me this woman joined the church more for the support and friendship she needed rather than for any spiritual beliefs. Sadly she had become caught in her own trap to be victim to sustaining the pains by pacifying the values of the people she chose to be her friends. I do not know if her pains really returned. Was it a fib, a little white lie or make believe that amounts to no more than a harmless means to restore something that gave her the social support she so wanted?

This was a living example of how we all have a hand in making our destinies and futures by dint of what we choose to believe or to be fearful of.

THE HEALING POWER OF TOUCH AND A HUG

The simple transfer of a supporting energy in human or even animal touch is widely recognised, accepted indeed encouraged in many nursing and retirement homes. Hence the keeping of pets such as cats, dogs, birds, ponies or almost any animal, even snakes, rats, mice, spiders and many exotic creatures, all can have a subtle beneficial effect on our well-being. Of course that is depending on how we feel about certain animals. Just as many who adore cats and dogs, there are those who just freeze at the sight or presence of these popular pets. That aside, the simple yet complex ability of an animal showing interest, seeking our protection and affection is certainly therapeutic. The amazing therapy of swimming with and touching dolphins is perhaps more widely acknowledged as something quite extraordinary and one many regard as having a deep and profound spiritual connection.

My own interpretation of this form of spirituality is the sense of feelings and awareness or belief that the dolphin understands, loves and enjoys swimming with humans. So that spirituality is actually the feeling of being accepted for exactly who we are; warts and all. This is something I recognise in my method of support healing. Because it focuses on non-interference, furthermore it is also none-judgemental. This particular connection with the animal world seems to be able to release within us a strong euphoric emotion, invariably described as a spiritual experience. How far this activity actually contributes to a healing process is difficult to assess but certainly it pleases Hippocrates, as there is little chance of it doing any harm.

On the basis the dolphins connect and do not interfere, then perhaps healing occurs at many different levels. However it is fairly clear these animal/human connections bound with mutual love and affection enables emotional barriers to melt away, thus giving way to renewed wellbeing. So many pet lovers are convinced beyond doubt that their close bonding with their pooches results in their better emotional and physical wellbeing and unconditional love.

Beyond this there is another issue of how a pet responds gently to one person and shows fear or acts in an aggressive way to another?

There are other mysteries of how animals know when we are in trouble emotionally or our lives are at risk? Why do they radically change their normal aggressive or wary behaviour to give us comfort or actively help our survival when normally they would keep their healthy self protective distance?

The answer is apparently in two parts. That of body language and the telepathic energy messages sent out automatically when we are in trouble. This is not simply between animals and humans. We all have experienced when others sense our troubled minds particularly when we knowingly send out silent telepathic calls for help. Because there are many recorded cases of animal acts of benevolence, indeed bravery, this suggests those animals will help both animals and humans when they are injured or in trouble. This is interesting as it indicates like humans, animals are able to break out of their normal fear instincts and quite incredibly put their own lives at risk to save another that is in mortal danger. All indication are that animals have retained a far better connection to their intuitive and telepathic intelligence and the field of energy and information than we humans. We have learnt to rely on written and vocal languages. In recent decades we have moved even further away from intuition and telepathy, largely due to the over use of the ubiquitous mobile telephone, computers and the internet to communicate. Hardly surprising the word spirituality is much used but little understood.

Feelings generally give clues to something we sense, where as intuition gives specific information. We do still use these subliminal communicating skills though we are far less conscious of doing so. Ulterior motives such as to manipulate, harm, kill or eat resonate with the animal world at a high level of awareness. Remember we are our thoughts so animals likely know the risks of our thoughts before we are fully aware of them ourselves. Talk to any experienced horse whisperer, they will confirm how these lines or fields of unspoken communication can either nurture or prevent any working contact across the species.

These observations demonstrate why as a support healer unconditional respect for the patient's innate healing intelligence is so important. I have no doubts the patient's subconscious intelligence, innate healing and all other centres of intelligence, including their

Survival and Self Protection intelligence knows a healer's true motivations and everything they are secretly thinking.

"I have never experienced anything so powerful." - "I have never been so emotionally touched." Or "Wow, that was incredible. – I feel so good I do not want to move. I fear I will wake up and lose this wonderful feeling."

The above are a few of the expressive words people have used to verbalise their inner feelings after support healing. These expressions are the same as those experiencing their feeling of unconditional love when swimming with, touching or hugging a dolphin. But what deeper understandings lie within those words, "powerful, emotionally touched, incredible or simply wow?" These words do not claim to be anything more than they are. Yet they represent a power, no more, no less than is needed so they are expressions of changes that something so small or so great has happened inside them. I came to be aware these words were inner expressions as though they can feel their body healing itself.

THE SPARK OF LIFE AND SPIRITUALITY

The spiritual issue related to the spark of life must have crossed the minds of most people. However, as the spark of life is so illusive any spiritual spark may yet prove to be another myth. Close to Geneva, Switzerland there is a twenty seven kilometres circular tunnel one hundred metres below the surface. It is full of high-tech equipment cumulatively referred to as a particle accelerator it is also known as the largest machine on this planet. That equipment is devoted to accelerating miniscule bits of matter and energy at enormous speeds and then crashing them into each other. The objective is to find what matter is made of also how those particles came into being. If scientists at the CERN Large Hadron particle collider close in on the physical and scientific truth of what has been described as the God factor, medical science may finally have a handle on what the spark of life really is all about and therefore improve medical and neuroscience understanding of how to preserve and nurture it far better than is being achieved so far.

I started out in a world of healing where words like God, spiritual guides or soul energy were scattered liberally by people who really believed they knew what they were talking about. All I had was a head full of questions and practically zero understanding of any sensible meaning of those words. The fact I was following my intuitive and telepathic intelligence, meant that although I had little conscious understanding of what I was really doing, that proved to be perfect. Apart from the odd occasions when I began interfering most of the time I was doing just fine.

Now I am more comfortable with medical and neuroscience and the science of the universe and crashing electrons into each other at incredible speeds in order for me to understand who I am, what makes me and my healing technique works. I am not frightened or offended should a team of scientists prove the God factor is a miniscule part of a particle, which needs a completely new language to begin to describe how it was created from stardust and now governs each one of us and for that matter also our entire universe and other galaxies far in the distance.

It only fills me with intrigue as I listen to scientists explaining how thousands of black holes or accumulations of dark matter many light years away from planet Earth are now believed to be the very engines that make our world and each one of us possible. If so, those black holes may just prove to be the origin of the God factor although the same question raises its head. How did they come into being? Given they are themselves many light years across, it may be wiser to stick to focusing our attention on what the spark of life really is rather than how it was created. Whatever one feels or believes about this particular science, none of it detracts from the fact we are and will always be matter, energy, form and incredible amounts of information governed by centres of intelligence, feelings, beliefs and emotions.

Whatever spirituality means, the fact is it is a broad concept of many meanings, myths, perceptions, perspectives, assumptions, aspirations and beliefs. The spark of life seems to universally include a sense of connection to something bigger than ourselves and all our combined beliefs. We may be aware of whatever this is but being ultimately unexplainable; we are nonetheless evidence that it has a place and meaning in our lives. We only have difficulty to describe it because we cannot see it or touch it because it is either too big or too small. Ultimately we are left with solely the capability to sense ours and others sparks of life. Is this the point that ancient theorists created the presumption of the existence of a God?

Researching this concept, I find it typically involves a search for meaning in life and of life. As such, it is a universal human experience, thus we return to the spark of healing and all that any healing is all about. Dogma does not appear to have any great impact on the fact of the spark of life perhaps because no one knows what it is. We the masses become convinced by experiential logic that our only hope of hanging onto it all making some sort of sense is to attach it to one fundamental belief in an intelligent maker. For believers this belief is somehow related to the creation of a God. That is even though this God is ultimately indefinable by any scientific reasoning. This raises the question of who or what created God. For non-believers the spark of life is undeniable and since other peoples' God seems to care nothing for the spark of life they have no need for such a heartless God. Is this where Jesus fits into the picture as a co-star to plug this gaping hole by injecting the prospects and benefits of love, peace and caring into our lives?

Every atom and molecule in this and all other universes have intelligence and that intelligence is what the scientists are doing their best to understand through science rather than through assumptions, myths, stories, hearsay and spirituality. This does not change human beings, humanity, or the meaning of life. It does not change healing and the subconscious centres of intelligence within the brain and body. It would not change the remotest part of spirituality because until we understand how the very first spark of life was formed, spirituality remains a search for meaning in our lives, therefore a function of mind and unique individual perception. The paradox is the day scientists bust the myth and are 100% certain that life is created in a cloud of dark matter, then spirituality will be stronger than ever. This is because those in need of finding God will all turn their heads to our galaxy's Milky Way in search of the particular black hole and dark matter where they will be certain to find God, Jesus, heaven and very possibly also paradise.

As we see from artists, musicians, inventors and story writers, these things also make our world go around in another way and another language. We can be spiritual creatures looking for meaning in fleeting experiences we may describe as uplifting. One journalist said when seeing one of the two large Hadron particle accelerators at the CERN installation, *"it is the most beautiful thing I have ever seen."*

To stand in that great cathedral of science in action, I have no doubt that journalist's comment was as much a spiritual moment as it was an adrenalin rush. So which came first? Well emotional intelligence and a burst of adrenalin certainly came long after the first spark of life. Therefore, spirituality seems to be a product of needing to believe in an intelligence bigger than ourselves and therefore to understand what drives our emotional intelligence.

The truth of how we help ourselves by being generous in loving ourselves in the right way is seen in the above as it is in so many other ways. For me the neuroscience of innate healing intelligence is something quite tangible. When blocked and then freed to come back to life it is something awesome and so beautiful to experience. Like making an intricate watch or the biggest and complex machine in the world, success is in getting the right bits of the healing process in the right order at the right time so they can do their intended job in the most supreme harmony.

The fact is that whatever the origins of spirituality, it is the quality and sustainability of the information from it that counts. This is actually driving our need to find answers to the most ethereal of questions. This concerns where we come from, who or what the puppet master is and how he, she or it pulls our strings. What is our purpose for being here and the most sought after answer is what happens next. Because spirituality is steeped in a need to know it becomes clear how centuries ago as faith and therefore also emerging spirituality became entangled in alternative healing in search of answers and thus became known as spiritual or faith healing.

A sobering thought but one dear to me is that whatever the source of healing, it is "about being brutally honest." That means it either works, it seems to work for a short while or it really does not work at all. If it works that means there has been the right support with no well meaning interference. If the healing seems to work at least for a short time, then the support was in reality unnecessary interference. If the healing does not work then there has been no support and the emotional intelligence is still blocked.

But let us remember we should remain vigilant if we are not privy to the reasons why or when healing begins working. This is of course because healing will only work when the owner of the inner healer is emotionally, consciously and subconsciously ready to allow it to work. There is no doctor, surgeon, therapist or support healer on this earth that has the capability or right to know such things. We must remember the most fundamental oath of all forms of healers in, "The Spark of Life is the ultimate intelligence so, be guided by it, do not interfere and do no harm. Always be aware of its presence, endeavour to support it by whatever means is appropriate and never interfere unless guided by brutally honest and genuine squeaky clean telepathy and intuition."

Chapter 19

IT'S ALL IN THE MIND

M edical research and sciences are capable of seeing deep inside the body even inside individual cells. It is possible to observe the brain interior as the creation of thoughts and ideas form and travel to other regions of the brain.
Dr. Deepak Chopra's said (Chopra Deepak, 1998):
"Intelligence is more important than the matter of the body, since without it, that matter would be undirected, formless and chaotic."

At the age of eight, long before I knew anything about healing, I had watched my own father in the last throws of dying of lung cancer. I saw the destructive results of radiation treatment of the early 1950's. I witnessed how the radiation visibly burnt his skin and how the cancer slowly but surely whittled his body away until there was nothing to sustain his Spark of Life.

Chemotherapy, radiation treatment and medical science has come a long way since the 1950s. In those days doctors understood that they had to stop rogue cells from dividing and the best way to do that was to destroy them with radiation. What the doctors did not understand was why healthy cells turn into cancerous cells. That was until 2007. Here is part of a medical research note published in November 2007 by Dean Felsher MD PhD associate professor of medicine (Oncology) and of pathology at the Stanford University School of Medicine. It illustrates in different words exactly as I have described in the above chapters.

Quote: *"Our research implies that by shutting off a critical cancer gene, tumour, cells can realise that they are broken and restore this physiological fail-safe program."*

This is to say; "(*shutting off a critical cancer gene, tumour cells)*" means shutting down damaging chaotic self destructive cell behaviours, which maintains the cancer growth. (*"Can realise that they are broken and restore physiologic fail-safe program)"* is the psycho-cybernetic process in action at the cellular level. This is a similar principle as in the case of AIDS, where normal blood "T" cells are unable to recognise the virus as alien; therefore they cannot alert the "killer T cells" to attack the AIDS virus. In simple language, the innate healing system does not know there is a problem. What I understand from this is that my father did not die from cancer he was killed by the destructive effects of radiation treatment long before the cancer would have ended his life. The collateral damage was so great; he had no remaining immune system and innate healing defences to sustain his spark of life.

The connection with the above and the law of psycho-cybernetic intelligence is that it is only possible to keep on a desired course so long as you have some means of knowing you are veering off course. By definition that means you have to poses a means of realising you are off course. This is the reason for the feedback, but if that part is not working, then as in the case of AIDS and cancers, the body is on a course to long term disaster. Chemotherapy and radiation aim to do this by killing cancerous cells. These are very blunt instruments that destroy the bad the ugly and the good. Worse still the effect is to scatter rogue information throughout the body, which appear as secondary early formation tumours. When surgeons find this state is when they know that for them it is game over.

The fact that cancer cells are able to develop unchallenged is because the innate healing systems intelligence is essentially blocked. This may be because the cancerous cells are the same matter and substance. The fact their information program is still intact but switched off, may be the reason the innate healing systems intelligence does not register there is something wrong and thus does not release its own dogs of war defence systems.

Nonetheless, the above quote from Professor Felsher and the following additional information are all important links that helped me with more understanding of how my support healing gift worked.

Medical awareness of apoptosis and senescence programs and emotional intelligence are the key to answering the question of how does support healing support the patient's innate healing intelligence to heal cancers. The truth has to be in not killing cancer cells because that does too much collateral damage and defeats the real healer. Is this a better solution to understand how to switch on again those cell senescence programs? Thus in one go completely bypassing the need to kill any cell let alone cause so much additional and unnecessary damage to the patient. This answer is the epitome of Hippocrates' warning to do no harm. As I explained in the earlier chapters the healer's principle roll is to be available so the patient's innate healing system intelligence can copy the vital information it needs to restart those pesky cell senescence programs.

Prof. Felsher also said; *"What was unexpected was just the fact that cancer cells had retained the ability to undergo senescence at all."* This is the aging process which works alongside apoptosis or programmed cell death. Professor Felsher also said: *"Our research implies that by shutting off a critical cancer gene, tumour cells can realise that they are broken and restore this physiologic fail-safe program,"*

Cancer researchers had long thought the senescence and apoptosis mechanism had to be irreversibly disrupted or destroyed for a cancer tumour to develop into what is called a state of immortality. Felsher described senescence as acting as a fail-safe mechanism to stop cancer.

"When a 'T' cell detects a deleterious mutation, it launches the senescence process, resulting in the permanent loss of the cell's ability to proliferate, thus halting any cancer."

As the above was taken out of an extended text, I will clarify that "*(the cancer cell's ability to proliferate)*" refers to a cell's senescence (aging) program being turned off thus reaching this state referred to as immortality. Without senescence and with no limitations the cancer cells continue to divide uncontrolled.

"Resulting in the permanent loss of the cell's ability to proliferate, thus halting any cancer." Refers to reactivating the senescence program, which means the cells can die and that blocks cancerous cells from dividing in their chaotic uncontrolled form. (Felsher, 2007) The above quote taken from FierceBioResearcher publication 07.31.07

Consequently, the conclusion is my healing gift notably via a telepathic transfer of vital information appears to have had the ability to raise the alarm within the immune system allowing it as Felsher described, *"to reactivate or restore this physiologic fail-safe program."* Once the cancerous cells had been blocked from dividing or repeating themselves, it seemed the innate healing intelligence was able to carry out additional necessary healing under its own steam.

Is this the key to all therapy, healing and orthodox medicine that works? Whether intentional or not it can be said that all medicine works with the mind and body/mind systems. If those systems fail, no amount of medical treatment can turn a moribund body protective system into a live healthy being unless there is sufficient internal direction to cause it to do so.

Dr. Deepak Chopra says, *"without the right information,* (i.e. DNA and senescence programs of information) *cells are just uncontrollable matter."* This is to say the immune system and innate healing system and every cell in the body are at risk of losing the battle of life the moment they lose the right information that keeps them on song and on message with their spark of life program.

This takes knowing ourselves to a completely different level. It opens the door to understanding the importance of loving and respecting ourselves right down to the cellular level. This is the master key and doing everything possible to support in a positive way, while also avoid doing ourselves any invisible harm. Thus we need the ideal values, disciplines and self-leadership to fulfil this most important task of helping our innate healing systems intelligence to remain on song.

Healing someone's cancer as an alternative healer may be scorned at by professionals or seen by believers as a remarkable event, a miracle of faith or spiritual intervention. I understand this concept although I believe it is utterly misguided and largely for a lack of understanding how the brain and body works also how it manages and heals itself on a 24/7continual basis. I believe the essence of my theory for why my healing method works, has gone some way to indicating the key to curing cancer is as much related to neuroscience as it is to medical science.

The body's innate healing system intelligence realising something is broken, not working or switched off is an issue that frequently comes up in the complications of the body's self healing capability. To shed more light on the intelligence aspect of healing, I refer to a time when I was called to a London children's hospital to help a young boy who would not respond to the vital dialysis he needed. I was shown to his bedside but hardly could see him for the tubes and wires attached to his body and machines festooned around him. I was not allowed to get close to his bed for contamination reasons.

With my knowledge and experience of telepathy and distance healing also support healing on the hoof, I made contact with his innate healing intelligence from where I stood some yards from his bed. Despite the complications, I sensed the telepathic connection with the boy's subconscious intelligence. I waited for the usual signal that I had done all I could and then left the hospital. The next morning I received a telephone call to say the boy was making a rapid recovery. The dialysis along with the appropriate medication spontaneously began to work and do their job soon after I left the hospital.

I like this case because as the boy was in a semi-coma state. Normally the patient's consent is vital if only to get access. Being in a semi-coma the boy's permission was impossible by verbal means. This hurdle was overcome as part of my telepathic connection includes the act of offering my support and assurance there will be no interference and finally asking for guidance as to what is required. In addition, this case appears to be a situation of alternative support healing working with and alongside orthodox medicine without any special arrangement. It reminds me of so many accounts of surgeons and doctors who knew they could do no more and thereafter the outcome was up to the patient and their innate healing system. This recognition is important because it points to healing being a team game.

The innate healing systems intelligence is the important first line defence. Doctors, surgeons and hospitals are the second level of support. The evidence of so many of my support healing cases suggests that when both the above fail, support healing can be the crucial difference that unlocks the first line defence to do its own thing, also enabling the body to work with the second line defence, so the three combined make a significant difference.

Of course all the above is nothing but conjecture. Where is the proof other than the anecdotal evidence that the boy began a remarkable recovery after I departed? It is only the building of case histories like this that dependable patterns begin to emerge.

Having said all the above, there is a new treatment kid on the block and details of which I have just received. If the big pharmaceutics companies do not manage to block it by fair means or foul, it is likely to cause some confusion in the treatment of many diseases including cancer. This is what Dr. Sears has to say about it.

Quote:

"America's #1 Cancer Hospital
Rejects Chemo?"

"Doctors at America's leading cancer hospital are bucking chemo for a breakthrough "cancer pill" — one that has no side effects, costs $1, and eradicates even so-called "incurable" cancers."

"Why are these doctors risking their professional livelihoods to save their patients' lives? Why is the same thing happening at leading institutions like Baylor and Johns Hopkins hospitals? And how can you access this treatment yourself, without a prescription?"

The above is all part of the growing interest by so many doctors to find medical treatments that "Do no Harm. I am sure there will be many more such developments in the future. Perhaps "Big Pharma" will one day realise there is a place for them to make their profits and work within this new trend rather than against it. This is not something for me to become directly involved in so the best I can suggest is anyone interested in this information should go to: alsearsmd@send.alsearsmd.com

Chapter 20

FAITH

It is said that faith can move mountains. Also that faith can strike fear and doubt from our hearts. Perhaps it is important to remember that faith can be a double edged sword. In my experience; at its best; true sustainable faith is really one word that encapsulates experience, knowledge, understanding and personal leadership. The greater these qualities are; the greater the faith we have in ourselves or indeed something or someone else within which we propose to place our trust.

The personal leadership element is the vital process capable of knitting all the other factors into one reliable and sustainable faith. Now if we have the skills to add intuition and telepathy on demand into that mix, like a steroid booster, this supercharges our faith in ourselves and our capabilities. The net result is this potent mixture opens the way for us to do the seemingly impossible as if it was a stroll in the park.

When faith is supported by these verifiable facts; yes; it can produce miraculous results. Because blind faith out of dogma is self limiting, suppositions, misinformation and false gossip may let us down badly but do we really notice that? One of the strange characteristics of all faith guidance of this type is when they fail to perform they are immediately forgotten and rarely held to account. Only in extreme situations of entire villages collapsing after an earthquake, huge mud slides after torrential rain and families literally ripped apart by war, do we see men and women alike questioning their faith to explain why their God has so heartlessly abandoned and forgotten them.

Analysis of my personal self-healing experience led me to believe that a patient's persistent or serious illnesses are much to do with the behaviours, beliefs and attitudes automatically consciously and subliminally used to limit themselves.

Dr. Wiley became a specialist in healing arthritis because he suffered with this affliction himself. Much in the line of Dr Al Sears approach to medicines, Dr. Wiley set himself the task of finding a better solution than dangerous medications. After suffering his own body's arthritis earthquakes and tsunami catastrophes, he had lost faith in the accepted medical opinions of treating this condition.

Much in the same style, from a very young age I suffered with chronic hay-fever that plagued my life for a minimum six months of the year. That was from beginning of April to end August at the minimum. After years of treatment, tests and pills I was not much better so I lost trust in the medical system. Like Dr Wiley I began looking for better solutions and those turned out to be developing a faith by deed of experience, understanding and personal discipline and knowledge to find what my hay fever was all about.

Just as Dr. Wiley had found with arthritis, I discovered my hay-fever was due to self-limiting behaviours, which I knew nothing about albeit the signs were there. Then I realised it was possible to self improve my situation by ending the damage I had previously and unknowingly been doing to myself. This was wrapped up in misinformation style faith in the benefits of certain staple foods proclaimed to be healthy and nourishing. Now, almost fifty years later, doctors and nutritionists are guiding their patients to take similar actions. We all know about gluten in breads, then it became apparent that bakers yeasts were also problem. I was testing gluten free and yeast free breads but still suffered allergy reactions. I concluded there had to be something else in the grain that was contributory to an allergy reaction. This was dismissed politely as my imagination. Lo and behold as I am finishing this book I have word from a pharmacist that yes researchers have found something of the nature I was convinced about. No doubt the world will hear more of this new discovery in due course.

Although the methods were simple and quite easy to follow, the fundamental issues were a little more complex and required me having faith in something that was verifiable. By testing these strategies and developing more reliable tests, I built experience, knowledge, understanding and the positive verifiable feedback results. The practical and sustainable faith I have developed, now pro-actively enables me to avoid harming my inner healing system. Now it does not have to protect itself or react by wasting vital energy in producing histamines and consequently the severely limiting symptoms recognised as hay fever.

Like hay-fever, arthritis, gouty arthritis and related health conditions, they are generally believed to be connected to inherited gene programs. This turns out to be not that simple and is just the beginning of the story and not the sole and definitive cause. Dr. Mark Wiley explains in his book "Arthritis Reversed" that faith in such beliefs being irreversible is absolutely wrong. Believing one is doomed to pain and powerful medications with unpleasant side effects; even premature death; is, as Dr. Wily says, "absolutely wrong. In his book he exposes some myths about treating arthritis. He also lays out practical and simple methods by, which one may directly reduce the cause of the arthritis without potentially dangerous medications and their side effects. Like so many other health conditions arthritis and its allied conditions are tied to excess body inflammation. I found this interesting as I had already discovered body inflammation was also the underlying support to maintaining my allergic hay-fever sensitivity.

Medical researchers are finding more and more evidence that inner body inflammation is possibly the greatest cause of many limiting health conditions. Understanding inflammation and what cases it, we have a window into how to take personal control of our own innate healing system. This shows why it is important to understand what we are doing to ourselves, our health and comfort that is so wrong. In a nutshell, reduce the self limiting behaviours that cause inflammation we reduce the pain or stop the arthritis, hay-fever and a multitude of other health conditions, for which the pharmaceutical industry holds millions of people to ransom annually by selling unnecessary and expensive remedies.

In order to put a little flesh on these bones of advice, perhaps I should explain a little more. Reducing and managing body inflammation is largely to do with our thinking process, beliefs, values and mainly concerns unreliable faith in what we eat and drink. This is largely because we take what we are taught without taking notice and having faith in the feedback our body's are giving us.

Earlier I mentioned negative faith occurring in some of my patients. The reason for this was in the fact of orthodox medicine having failed them. Doctors and hospitals are the 'go to' place for medical help. For most people, when those fail, what is there to do but search for alternative options? Therefore, we no longer know what to believe or have faith in.

Some people go to extreme lengths, refusing to give up. As I mentioned one woman in Oslo went to three different specialists and then proceeded to take daily all their combined prescribed treatment. I said because she vomited all that medication she probably saved her own life. This void is equally likely to be filled by listening to and trusting in gossip, hearsay, grabbing at straws, any straws of hope no matter how contradictory. Some of those are frankly bizarre and others are downright fraudulent. Thus, it was clear to me how many patients had more faith in alternative, faith and spiritual healing not working but nonetheless until its all over, their thinking was why not give it a try as a long shot.

I discovered the above because I always asked about what alternative therapies my patient's had tried. I would never give advice but I did explain the difference in my support healing and how I believed it worked. This should not be dismissed, even so, many who arrived with a self limiting attitude were among those on the list of successes but then also they were the greatest convertees. This was because my support healing first supported them in dealing with the primary problem of self limiting faith, emotional issues like things that had been worrying them for years but, which they feared to properly deal with.

This invariably turned to my natural and intuitive form of life coaching, which was not interfering but supporting with verifiable information. Having helped them to fill in an understanding gap, this usually lifted a great stress weight from their minds. Although proceeding with the support healing, I believe after the life coaching stage they were probably already healing themselves without the real need for any more support from me.

So anything other than substantiated, verifiable facts this leaves ad hock faith being no more than a mixture of pseudo-rational and irrational thinking based on dogma, hearsay, fear, doubt and baseless assumptions. I fully appreciate this conclusion is likely to offend many people. All I can say is examine what we have faith in with if necessary, brutal honesty and find all that is demonstrably reliable. Whatever is not demonstrably reliable then treat it with a healthy scepticism.

"The body must be credited with an immense fund of know-how."

Every person is unique. Do not take notice of what the masses say. Know yourself, test what you believe to be true for yourself, if it works for you with positive verifiable honest to goodness results then it is reasonable to have faith in it.

CONCLUSION.

The lessons of spontaneous support healing now seem almost yet not actually simple though it took many years to learn how they worked. Helping is what one considers to be the right thing to do but with a little or imperfect knowledge that can so often turn out to be counterproductive. As far as healing is concerned I believe this is best summed up as follows. "A little knowledge about activating someone else's spontaneous healing is a bad thing and trying to help or attempting to be the healer is even worse."

Everyone naturally wants to help someone in pain. The problem facing all support healers is that the brain, mind and body are so complex that in the context of support healing it is best to leave the healing to the intelligence that really does understand the problem, the perfect solution and really does know what it is doing.

Doctors, surgeons and hospitals are obviously vitally important and no healer can replace them. The problem is they do not have all the answers and some of the answers or drugs they resort to, do more damage, which in turn requires additional medication to heal the added problems. Therapeutic healers, which can include many therapies as well as NLP and life coaching, fit into the picture of healing both as a supplementary and an alternative support. One thing that does worry psychologists and some medical general practitioners is that so many of their patients may be treated more efficiently by NLP and life coaching therapy than orthodox medicine.

Clearly as I have explained in the above text, there are times when this superior intelligence does not recognise its system is in trouble. This is no time for alternative healers to fill the gap with what we believe is the ideal solution. The answer is to alert and support this intelligence so it can understand there is a problem. Then it can fix the blockage and then see the problem and heal it from the inside. Alternative healers must remain available as an external healing support but always avoiding any interference, thus letting the real healer do the real healing.

Bibliography mentioned within the above text.

Beilock, S. (n.d.). *Video: Human Brain: How Smart Can We Get?* *https://youtu.be/GxPWAw9nemU.* Chicago: University of Chicago.
Bethesda, (. (n.d.). Understanding Human Genetic Variation. *NIH Curriculum Supplement Series [Internet].Copyright © 2007-, BSCS. Bookshelf ID: NBK20363.*
Chopra Deepak, M. (1998). *Quantum Healing.* New York: Bantam Books ISBN: 0 553 17332 4.
Cook, G. (June 5 2012). Do Plants Think? *Scientific American.*
Daniel Chamovitz. (s.d.). *"What a Plant Knows,".* Tel Aviv.: Director of the Manna Center for Plant Biosciences at Tel Aviv University.
Denton, R. P. (2016). *High Performance After Burnout.* Geneva CH.: First House Press ISBN 9781512294705.
Dr Weil. Andrew, M. (s.d.). *Spontaneous Healing.* New York: Fawcett Columbine ISBN 0 449 91064 4.
Felsher, P. D. (2007, July 31). Senescence programming in cancerous cells. *FierceBioResearch.*
Gallwey, T. (2014). *The Inner Game of Golf.* New York: Pan MacMillian ISBN; 1447288475, 9781447288473.
Glouberman, D. D. (s.d.). *The Joy of Burnout.* London: Hodder Mobius ISBN: 0 340 82159 0.
Goleman, D. (1998). *Working with Emotional Intelligence.* New York: Bantum Books ISBN: 0 553 84023 0.
J. Allen Hobson, S. H. (1999). *States of Mind.* New York: The Dana Press ISBN: 0 471 39973 6.
Locke, D. C. (1987). *The Healer Within.* New York: Penguin Group Mentor ISBN:0 451 62554 4.
Schûzenberger, A. A. (1998). *The Ancestor Syndrome.* New York: Brunner-Routlage ISBN: 0 415 19187 4.
Spector, T. (2003). *Your Genes Unzipped.* London: Robson Books ISBN: 1 86105 662 1.
Wiley, Dr. Mark, *Arthritis Reversed.* ISBN. 978-0-615-97650-1

BIBLIOGRAPHY General reading of interest.

THE HEALER WITHIN The new medicine of mind and body
Steven Locke, M.D., and Douglas Colligan ISBN 0-451-62554-4
QUANTUM HEALING Exploring the frontiers of Mind/body Medicine
Deepak Chopra, M.D. ISBN 0-553-17332-4
STEVEN PINKER - HOW THE MIND WORKS.
Steven Pinker ISBN 0-140-24491-3
YOUR GENES UNZIPPED How your genetic inheritance shapes your life
Tim Spector ISBN 1-86105-662-1
THE ANCESTOR SYNDROME Transgenerational therapy and the hidden
links in the family tree Anne Ancelin Schûzenberger ISBN 0-415-19187-4
SPONTANEOUS HEALING How to discover and enhance your body's
natural ability to
maintain and heal itself.
Andrew Weil, M.D. ISBN: 0-449-91064-4
WORKING WITH EMOTIONAL INTELLIGENCE
Daniel Goleman ISBN 0-553-84023-1
PSYCHO-CYBERNETICS 2000
Maxwell Malts Foundation
Bobbe Sommer ISBN 0-13-263849-5
THE HUMAN MIND
Robert Winston ISBN 0-593-05210-2
THE ART OF LEADING YOURSELF Tap the power of your emotional
intelligence
Randi B. Noyes ISBN 0-09-188973-1
USE YOUR HEAD
Tony Buzan BBC ISBN 0-563-37103-X
SEVEN LIFE LESSONS OF CHAOS Spiritual wisdom from the science of
change
John Briggs & F. David Peat ISBN 0-06-093073-X
MIND MAGIC How to develop the 3 components of intelligence that matter
most in today's world
John Laurence Miller, Ph. D. ISBN 0-07-143320-1
PATTERNS OF THE HYPNOTIC TECHNIQUES OF MILTON
ERICKSON
Richard Bandler and John Grinder ISBN 091699001X
THE HEALING OF EMOTIONS Awakening the fearless self
Chris Griscom ISBN 0-553-40267-6

THE JOY OF BURNOUT How burning out unlocks the way to a better, brighter future.
Dr Dina Glouberman ISBN 0-340-82159-0
STOP THINKING START LIVING Discover lifelong happiness
Richard Charlson ISBN 0-7225-3547-3
THE SEVEN SPIRITUAL LAWS OF SUCCESS A practical guide to the fulfilment of your dreams.   Deepak Chopra ISBN 0-593-04083-X
THE PECKING ORDER Which Sibling succeeds and why
Dalton Conley ISBN 0-375-42174-2
SYSTEMS THINKING Essentials skills for creativity and problem solving
Joseph O'connor & Ian McDermott ISBN 0-7225-3442-6
THE POWER OF NOW How winning companies sense & respond to change using real time
technology. Vivek Ranadivé ISBN 0-07-135684-3
THE MINDMAP BOOK Radiant thinking. The major evolution in human thought
Tony Buzan ISBN 0-563-37101-3
FEEL THE FEAR AND DO IT ANYWAY by Susan Jeffers ISBN 0-09-9741100-8
THE POWER OF YOUR SUBCONSCIOUS MIND
Dr Joseph Murphy, D.R.S., Ph.D., D.D., L.L.D
ISBN 0-553-58318-2
PSYCHO CYBERNETICS 2
Paul G. Thomas ISBN 0-86332-898-9
Wiley, Dr. Mark, *Arthritis Reversed.* ISBN. 978-0-615-97650-1
Tambuli Media, www.TambuliMedia.com
THE INNER GAME OF GOLF
W. Timothy Gallwey ISBN 0-679-45760-7

www.ingramcontent.com/pod-product-compliance
Lightning Source LLC
Chambersburg PA
CBHW071412180526
45170CB00001B/84